国家级继续教育学习班培训教材

上海卫生系统先进适宜技术推广项目(编号:2013SY063)

上海市杨浦区人才专项发展基金(鼎元资金)高层人才科研成果转化类资金项目

AH-1型取石系统在膀胱结石治疗中的应用

主　编　李爱华

副主编　李威武　陆鸿海

　　　　张　峰　吴道忻

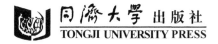

同济大学出版社
TONGJI UNIVERSITY PRESS

内 容 提 要

目前,泌尿外科尚缺乏能满意地用于治疗大体积膀胱结石的专用内镜。由本书主编李爱华医生研发的 AH-1 型取石系统为泌尿外科医生提供了一种集检查诊断、固定结石、提供碎石通道、冲吸碎石、回旋流自动收集碎石、抓取碎石和连续冲洗等功能为一体的多功能膀胱结石治疗内镜。解决了目前在经尿道治疗膀胱结石时只能使用其他替代内镜作为碎石平台的窘境。

本书从临床实践出发,结合国内外最新发展动态,概要介绍了膀胱结石形成的解剖、病理生理、病因学和流行病学基础,临床病史、体格检查、实验室检查、影像学检查、诊断注意事项和药物治疗方法等内容。重点介绍了现有手术方法、AH-1 型取石系统的技术方案、实验数据、临床用途,以及 AH-1 型取石系统经尿道治疗膀胱结石的规范化方案、与现有手术方法的临床疗效比较、治疗大体积膀胱结石的疗效等内容。

本书可供泌尿外科医生及相关专业人员作为及时了解膀胱结石基础知识和临床最新治疗进展的继续教育教材使用。

图书在版编目(CIP)数据

AH-1 型取石系统在膀胱结石治疗中的应用/李爱华主编.--上海:同济大学出版社,2017.1
ISBN 978-7-5608-6748-9

Ⅰ.①A… Ⅱ.①李… Ⅲ.①膀胱疾病-结石(病理)-诊疗 Ⅳ.①R694

中国版本图书馆 CIP 数据核字(2016)第 325298 号

AH-1 型取石系统在膀胱结石治疗中的应用

主编 李爱华

责任编辑 陈佳蔚 **责任校对** 徐春莲 **封面设计** 潘向蓁

出版发行　同济大学出版社　　　www.tongjipress.com.cn
　　　　　(地址:上海市四平路 1239 号 邮编:200092 电话:021-65985622)

经　销　全国各地新华书店
印　刷　虎彩印艺股份有限公司
开　本　787 mm×1 092 mm　1/16
印　张　8.25
字　数　165 000
版　次　2017 年 1 月第 1 版　　2017 年 1 月第 1 次印刷
书　号　ISBN 978-7-5608-6748-9

定　价　42.00 元

编 委 会

主 编 简 介

复旦大学外科学医学博士、主任医师。同济大学附属杨浦医院、上海市杨浦区中心医院泌尿外科主任、科研教学型副教授、博士生导师。从事临床医学和基础研究工作40年，重点领域为腔内微创治疗泌尿系结石、前列腺增生和泌尿系肿瘤。自1999年起，三次赴美国 Thomas Jefferson University Hospital 泌尿外科访问和博士后学习，师从国际著名教授 Demetrius H. Bagley 医生。原创技术 AH-1 型取石系统经尿道治疗膀胱结石术，2013年入选上海市卫生系统先进适宜技术推广项目，

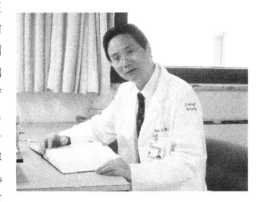

李爱华

并被国际泌尿外科学会(the Société Internationale d'Urologie)和国际泌尿外科疾病咨询委员会(International Consultation on Urological Diseases)联合编写的 *Stone Disease* 引用推荐。

目前担任中国医师协会男科分会男科医师培训委员会委员、上海市医学会泌尿外科专业委员会委员、上海市医学会男科专业委员会委员、上海市医学会男科专业委员会生殖器整形学组副组长、上海市泌尿外科会诊咨询服务部专家、上海市医疗技术临床应用能力评估专家库成员、上海市激光学会激光医学泌尿外科专业委员会委员。

1998年和2002年两次入选上海市区县卫生系学科带头人培养对象。上海市宝山区第四批专业技术拔尖人才、杨浦区第七批专业技术拔尖人才。

第一完成人获华夏医学科技奖三等奖1项、上海市技术发明三等奖1项、国家体育总局体育科技进步三等奖1项、上海市优秀发明选拔赛职工技术创新成果铜奖1项、上海市临床医疗成果三等奖1项、上海医学科技三等奖1项、上海市地区级科技进步奖4项。

第一完成人承担上海市科委课题1项、上海市卫生系统先进适宜技术推广项目1项、上海市卫生局科研课题3项、杨浦区人才发展专项资金(鼎元资金)资助高层次人才科研成果转化资金资助项目1项。

第一发明人获国际发明专利(PCT)1项、国家发明专利1项、实用新型专利6项。

第一作者和通讯作者国内外专业期刊发表学术论文123篇，其中SCI录用期刊23篇。

参编出版学术专著4种。在美国 Lippincott Williams & Wilkins 于2011年和2014年出版的第二版和第三版的 *The 5-Minute Urology Consult* 一书中担任国际编委。

序

    膀胱结石患者大多数是长期排尿不畅的老年前列腺增生患者或者是长期卧床的老年妇女。膀胱结石引起的临床症状通常会给这些患者带来极大的痛苦。经尿道碎石取石是治疗膀胱结石的最佳方法,但是目前国际上对于治疗多发性、大体积的膀胱结石,尚缺乏理想的专用内镜进行碎石和取石治疗。这些老年患者往往需要行开放手术进行取石治疗或腔内治疗。

    李爱华医生发明的 AH-1 型取石系统为临床泌尿外科医生提供了一种集固定结石、提供碎石通道、自动收集碎石、抓取碎石、冲吸碎石和连续冲洗等功能为一体的多功能内镜。尤其是术中固定结石后再碎石、回旋流自动收集碎石、镜鞘内一次抓取多枚碎石的技术和方法可缩短手术时间,提高碎石效率,拓展了内镜治疗膀胱结石的手术适应范围。李爱华医生的医疗团队在临床上已经通过这种微创腔镜手术方法有效地治疗了膀胱结石患者。在减轻患者痛苦的同时降低了患者的医疗负担,取得了良好的社会效益和经济效益。

    在国家级继续教育学习班教材的基础上,李爱华医生的团队参考、吸收了国外最新泌尿外科继续教育资料,认真编写了《AH-1 型取石系统在膀胱结石治疗中的应用》一书,详尽地介绍了膀胱结石的基础知识和治疗进展、AH-1 型取石系统的设计原理和临床功能、体外实验数据、临床应用方法、手术疗效和手术操作经验,并制定和介绍了操作规范化方案。

    本书内容全面、简洁明了,是一本有助于泌尿外科医生及时了解膀胱结石基础知识和临床最新治疗进展的继续教育教材。谨向从事泌尿外科工作的同道推荐本书。

(夏术阶)

2016 年 6 月

前　　言

在我国,膀胱结石多见于患有长期排尿困难疾病或长期卧床的老年患者,膀胱结石给老年患者的生活带来了极大的痛苦。目前,膀胱结石的常用治疗方法有:①膀胱切开取石术;②经皮膀胱造瘘碎石取石术;③经尿道膀胱碎石取石术。其中,膀胱切开取石术和经皮膀胱造瘘碎石取石术需要经腹部手术切口,创伤较大。经尿道碎石取石是最佳的微创治疗方法,但存在下述问题:①膀胱结石大且坚硬时,因膀胱空腔大,结石易滑动,不易被粉碎;②多发性结石或结石粉碎后形成的大量碎石因男性尿道长而弯曲,不易取出或取净;③经尿道反复取石易损伤尿道;④术中无法连续冲洗,手术视野不清;⑤膀胱壁充盈后变薄,容易损伤穿孔;⑥现有替代内镜设备较适用于直径小于 2 cm 的膀胱结石。因此,目前对于多发性、大体积的膀胱结石通常需要行开放手术进行治疗。

AH-1 型取石系统是一种基础型国际发明专利产品,经八年的设计和改进完善,现已由杭州时空候医疗器械有限公司批量生产。本系统具有独特的结构设计和手术功能。由窥镜、取石钳、碎石通道、镜桥、手柄、冲洗器、液体连续冲洗通道、镜鞘等构件组成。临床上解决了现有替代内镜治疗膀胱结石时存在的关键性和共性技术难题。可直视下经尿道进入膀胱,取石钳固定结石后再通过碎石通道用现有碎石设备进行碎石操作,大大提高了碎石效果。取石钳可利用回旋流自动收集碎石,然后在镜鞘内拉网摄取结石,一次可摄取多枚碎石,因此取石效率大幅提高。术中镜鞘内取石和采用冲吸器冲吸较多细小碎石,有效避免了反复经尿道取石对尿道黏膜的损伤。该系统具有连续冲洗功能,术中可保持视野清晰,不易误伤膀胱黏膜,能有效缩短碎石和取石的手术时间。经多中心应用已成功治疗 600 余例膀胱结石患者,其中大于 3 cm 的结石占 22%,最大结石为 6.6 cm,数目最多的病例为 172 枚 0.5~1.5 cm 结石。对于伴有的前列腺增生可同时实施经尿道前列腺切除术。

我国随着社会的老龄化,近年来膀胱结石发病率呈现稳定增长的趋势。应用 AH-1 型取石系统实施经尿道膀胱结石碎石取石术可避免或大大减轻手术创伤对老年患者产生的医源性创伤和痛苦,缩短康复时间,这符合医学伦理学和卫生经济学原则。

研发 AH-1 型取石系统的初衷是为了向泌尿外科临床医生提供一种能有效用于治疗膀胱结石的多功能内镜。经市卫计委和国家卫计委批准,先后多次主办了市级和国家级继续教育项目"AH-1 型取石系统的研发和临床应用"学习班。为此,与科室同事们一起编写了用于"AH-1 型取石系统经尿道治疗膀胱结石"的继续教育学习班教材,以供学员学习参考之用。在此基础上,我们又参考、吸收了国外泌尿外科继续教育资料,进行了认真的编写整理。希望通过本书的出版,能不辜负上级领导对我们的希望和支持,能有效地促进 AH-1 型取石系统经尿道碎石术这一中国原创技术在国内外得以广泛推广,同时能抛砖引玉,促进医疗器械国产化的进程。

在此,由衷地感谢中华泌尿外科学会主任委员孙颖浩院士、中国男科医师协会会长夏术阶教授、江西省泌尿外科学会主任委员王共先教授、浙江省泌尿外科学会主任委员谢立平教授、中华泌尿外科学会泌尿系结石专业委员会委员程跃教授,以及上海卫计委科研处和上海市泌尿外科学会的各位领导和老师对于这项工作的鼓励、支持和帮助。

由于编者才学疏浅,若有不尽完善之处,敬请各位老师和同行们不吝赐教。

李爱华

2016 年 12 月

目　　录

第一节
膀胱结石概况

膀胱结石是指存在于膀胱(或代膀胱的储尿囊)内的石头或钙化物。膀胱结石的生成通常与患者存在的尿液潴留有关。生成膀胱结石的原因有泌尿系统解剖异常、尿道狭窄、尿路感染、膀胱内异物等,但是膀胱结石也可发生在一些并不存在上述诱因的健康者身上。膀胱结石不一定是来源于上尿路的结石。目前,虽然西方国家膀胱结石的发病率较低,但是膀胱结石可引起患者产生特别严重的临床症状和明显的不适。

在全球范围内,儿童膀胱结石的发病率正缓慢下降,甚至在膀胱结石的高发区亦是如此。这主要归根于儿童营养状况的改善,孕期及产后的良好护理,以及对可引起膀胱结石疾病的重视和认识。预期儿童膀胱结石的发病率在21世纪将会得到进一步的下降,因此膀胱结石将逐步成为一种成人疾病。

采用 α 受体阻滞剂和 5α 还原酶抑制剂可以有效地改善前列腺增生患者的下尿路症状,促进膀胱的排空,降低膀胱结石的发病率。而去除膀胱结石的方法也已逐渐转变为微创手术治疗,从而明显降低了患者的住院时间和恢复时间。随着手术器械的不断改进和结石体积的不断缩小,微创手术碎石效果获得了不断的改善,因此,最终微创手术将可以完全替代开放手术进行膀胱结石的治疗。

一、解剖

前列腺体积增大是引起男性膀胱出口梗阻的主要解剖学原因。前列腺围绕着膀胱颈部呈现指环样生长,当体积增大时,可严重阻碍尿液排出。尿液潴留后,结晶物可在尿液中不断析出,进而形成结石。

女性患者的排尿功能障碍和尿潴留较少引起膀胱结石的生成。诱发膀胱结石生成的主要解剖因素包括膀胱憩室、阴道突出或尿道手术后的尿潴留加重。较少情况下,未能排出膀胱的物体被钙化后最终也会形成膀胱结石。

二、病理生理

大多数膀胱结石生成于膀胱内,还有部分膀胱结石起源于肾脏。它们初始时可以是一块脱落的 Randall 钙斑或蜕落的乳头黏膜,然后通过输尿管进入到膀胱内,随着尿液结晶的不断沉积,形成结石并不断增大。

但是,大多数体积较小的肾结石,可以在通过输尿管进入膀胱后,再依赖正常的膀胱收缩功能,通过没有梗阻的尿道排出体外。在老年男性患者中,尿酸成分的膀胱结石多在膀胱内生成,而草酸钙成分的结石通常是在肾脏形成。

成年人最常见的膀胱结石是尿酸结石,占 50% 以上。其次为草酸钙结石、磷酸钙结石、尿酸铵结石、半胱氨酸结石和磷酸镁铵结石。磷酸镁铵结石的形成通常与感染有关[1, 2]。但是令人奇怪的是,膀胱尿酸结石的患者往往并没有高尿酸血症或痛风病史。在多数病例中,膀胱结石的核心是一种化学成分,而结石的外层则是由多种化学物质组成。脊柱损伤患者伴发的结石通常是由磷酸镁铵或磷酸钙组成。

儿童患者中,膀胱结石的成分主要有磷酸铵结石,草酸钙结石或尿酸铵、草酸钙和磷酸钙混合结石[3]。在儿童膀胱结石高发地区,结石的高发与母乳和精制大米喂养有关。这些饮食中磷含量较低,从而导致氨分泌增高。通常,这些患儿可能摄入了较多的富含草酸的蔬菜,这会增加草酸结晶尿。这些患儿也可能摄入了较多的低柠檬酸的动物性蛋白膳食[3-5]。

膀胱结石可以是单发,也可以是多发,特别是有膀胱憩室时更易多发。膀胱结石的体积可以较小,也可以大到充满整个膀胱。结石的质地软硬不定。有些结石表面很光滑,也有些粗糙不平。一般情况下,膀胱结石可以在膀胱内随意滚动。但有时膀胱结石也会固定在膀胱内,如缝线残端和乳头状瘤表面钙化形成的结石或者膀胱内残留导管形成的结石。

在小儿膀胱结石高发地区,膀胱结石多见于 11 岁以下贫困人群的男孩,膀胱结石的发生与肾结石无相关性。相对于上尿路结石,治愈后的复发率较低[6]。

三、病因学

成年人引发膀胱结石的最常见病因是膀胱出口梗阻。前列腺增大、膀胱颈部抬高、残余尿过多都可形成尿液潴留,继而尿液结晶沉淀形成核心,并不断增大,最终导致结石的生成。此外,尿潴留容易引发尿路感染,进一步促进膀胱结石的生成。

一项长达 8 年以上有关出现神经源性膀胱的脊髓损伤患者的随访研究发现,36%的脊髓损伤者伴发膀胱结石。随后的研究报告提示,脊髓损伤患者的良好护理可使膀胱结石发生率下降到 10%以下。在一项针对 93 例脊髓损伤伴发膀胱结石患者的回顾性研究中,Bartel 等人发现,长期留置导尿比间歇性导尿或反射性排尿具有更高的膀胱结石发生率和复发率[7]。

放射性或血吸虫病性膀胱炎也会诱发膀胱结石[8]。放疗引起的膀胱和前列腺损伤可导致组织退化形成钙化灶,这些病灶进而形成膀胱结石的核心。先天性或后天性膀胱憩室可以引起尿液残留,继而导致结石生成。其他可引起尿潴留及促进膀胱结石生成的解剖因素包括疝内容物为膀胱的腹股沟滑疝[9]。

膀胱扩大术后的小儿患者产生膀胱结石的原因是多方面的。Mathoera 等人在一项 89 例膀胱扩大术后并发膀胱结石的小儿患者研究中发现,泄殖腔畸形、阴道重建、输尿管再植、膀胱颈部手术是诱发膀胱结石生成的重要原因[10]。预防性使用抗生素可治疗反复出现的尿路感染,从而降低磷酸镁铵结石的形成,但是并不能明显减少膀胱结石的总发生率。

引起膀胱结石生成的其他病因还有膀胱异物,异物可以成为结石形成的核心。根据膀胱异物的来源又可分为医源性异物和非医源性异物。医源性异物包括缝线、破损的气囊导尿管、气囊导尿管表面形成的蛋壳样钙化物、缝合钉、输尿管支架、移入的避孕器、手术植入残留物以及前列腺尿道支架等[11-15]。缝线可诱发膀胱结石。如果是突入膀胱腔内的缝线引起的膀胱结石,则早期就可出现明显的临床症状。相反,膀胱壁内缝线腐烂诱发的膀胱结石,则临床症状出现得较晚[16]。非医源性异物包括患者为寻求娱乐和各种其他原因置入膀胱腔内的物体[17]。

尿流改道术后患者的代谢异常不是引起膀胱结石的重要原因。这些患者的结石成分主要是钙和磷酸镁铵。在罕见的病例中,药物如病毒蛋白酶抑制剂等可能是形成膀胱结石的来源[18]。

Childs 等在一项回顾性研究中对照分析发现,57 例前列腺增生导致膀胱出口梗阻的手术患者中 27 例伴有膀胱结石。这些伴发膀胱结石的患者大多有肾结石和痛风病史,24 h 尿液检查发现,尿液 pH 值和镁浓度偏低,而尿酸含量过高。提示包括代谢因素在内的多种因素共同导致了膀胱结石的形成[19]。

总之,在美国或者欧洲生活的健康者被诊断为膀胱结石,通常会进行全面的泌尿系统检查,以查明引起尿液潴留的原因。常见的诱发因素包括前列腺增生、尿道狭窄、神经源性膀胱、膀胱憩室、输尿管脱垂等先天性畸形和膀胱颈部挛缩。女性患者则包括尿失禁修复吊带过紧、膀胱膨出和膀胱憩室[20]。

四、流行病学

19 世纪以来,随着饮食结构的改善和尿路感染的有效控制,美国和西欧地区的原发性膀胱结石发病率呈逐年显著下降的趋势。同时,这些国家的儿童膀胱结石发病率也在持续下降。目前在西半球,膀胱结石主要发生在 50 岁以上伴有膀胱出口梗阻的男性患者。

但是膀胱结石发病率在欠发达国家和地区,如泰国、缅甸、印度尼西亚、中东及北非地区仍然维持在较高水平。在这些地区,膀胱结石发病率虽有所下降,但依然是影响儿童健康的一种疾病。其中男性儿童的发病率远高于女性儿童[21]。

1977 年,Van Reen 出版了一本有关特发性膀胱结石专题的论文集[5]。很遗憾,主要是由于发展中国家和地区医院的记录资料不全,因此无法准确计算出世界各国和地区膀胱结石的发病率,不能精确绘制出膀胱结石发病率的世界分布图。虽然在一些膀胱结石高发国家进行了一些调查研究,但是获得的调查结果并不一致。

五、病史和体格检查

膀胱结石患者可以没有任何症状，也可以出现下述系列症状，如耻骨上区腹痛、排尿困难、间歇性排尿、尿频、排尿踌躇、夜尿增多和尿潴留等[2]。膀胱结石患儿的家长往往主诉患儿有阴茎异常勃起和间断性遗尿[8]。

其他常见的症状还有终末肉眼血尿、伴随不同程度疼痛的排尿突然中断，疼痛可放射到阴茎、阴囊、会阴、后背及臀部。这种不适可以是钝痛或锐痛，也可以因为运动或者突然的体位动作而加重。采用仰卧位、俯卧位或者头低侧卧位都可以使得原本嵌顿于膀胱颈部的结石返回膀胱内，从而减轻疼痛。

膀胱结石的非特有症状包括镜下或肉眼血尿、脓尿、菌尿、结晶尿，尿液培养有分解尿素的微生物生长。

应仔细询问患者是否有盆腔手术史，特别应注意是否有人工合成物的置入病史[22]。

体检时常见的阳性体征包括耻骨上区饱满、压痛，如果患者伴有急性尿潴留，可以在耻骨上区触及膨大的膀胱。女性患者的常见体征包括膀胱膨出、尿流改道后的吻合口狭窄和神经源性膀胱患者的神经功能障碍。

早期膀胱结石的诊断是由经尿道途径的 van Buren 声波进行的。van Buren 声波接触结石后可引起声波传导杂音或震动，以此确定结石的存在。随着膀胱镜技术的不断改进，这种诊断方法如今已不再使用了。

目前，腹部盆腔 X 线平片已被广泛用于诊断非透光性结石。但是以尿酸为主要成分的结石是透光性结石，除非还包有钙化的外壳，否则 X 线片很难显示这类结石。膀胱镜检查、平扫 CT、超声成像等方法已广泛应用于膀胱结石的诊断[8]。

六、诊断注意事项

膀胱内需要鉴别诊断的移动性充盈缺损包括血块、真菌球、带蒂的乳头状尿路上皮癌。需要鉴别诊断的非移动性充盈缺损还包括尿路上皮癌、血块、结石。

七、实验室检查

尿液分析，廉价、快速，并可提供有价值的信息。膀胱结石患者尿液检查时，亚硝酸盐、白细胞酯酶和血尿测试结果可呈阳性。膀胱结石常会引起排尿困难和尿痛，因此患者每天会减少液体摄入量，导致尿比重增高。成人膀胱尿酸结石患者尿液 pH 值可呈酸性。显微镜检查时可发现红细胞和脓尿，尿液中的微小结晶体形态通常与结石成分一致。

尿液细菌培养＋药敏检查，尿培养有助于确定敏感药物，指导相关的抗感染治疗。

全血细胞计数检查，膀胱出口梗阻伴感染的患者白细胞计数升高并有左移。

全面的代谢功能测定，膀胱出口梗阻患者肌酐水平可升高。

其他的检查结果，可能会显示潜在的异常。

八、放射线检查

影像学检查的首选项目是肾、输尿管、膀胱平片（KUB），这是最廉价和最易获取的放射线检查。单独拍摄或作为静脉肾盂造影检查（IVP）的第一张片子的KUB 可用于检查非透光性结石。纯尿酸和尿酸铵结石是透光性结石，但可被一层不透光的钙化沉积物包裹，常见有层叠状结构。这些变化与代谢、感染和周期性血尿状况有关[8]。

对于初始检查 KUB 阴性而不能排除结石的患者应进行膀胱超声检查，其可对结石、肿瘤和血凝块进行鉴别诊断。膀胱造影或 IVP 检查时，膀胱结石通常显示为膀胱内有充盈缺损。

检查时，随体位变动的充盈缺损多为膀胱结石，鉴别诊断对象包括血凝块、真菌球和带蒂乳头状尿路上皮癌。不随体位变动的充盈缺损，可能是附着于膀胱壁的缝线结石或憩室内结石，鉴别诊断包括尿路上皮癌、血凝块和结石。IVP

也可用于诊断相关的病因,如上尿路结石、输尿管脱垂、膀胱膨出、前列腺增生和膀胱憩室等[8]。

九、超声检查

随着超声检查的日益普及,这种廉价快速的诊断方法已被广泛地使用于膀胱结石的诊断。超声检查通常显示结石后方有经典的声影,超声检查能有效地识别透光和不透光的结石[23]。

十、CT 检查

通常因其他原因,如腹痛、盆腔肿块或怀疑脓肿等可进行 CT 扫描,在不用静脉注射造影剂时,平扫 CT 也可显示膀胱结石。非增强螺旋 CT 扫描对诊断泌尿结石具有高度的敏感性和特异性。即使是纯尿酸结石也可用这项检查确诊。在使用造影剂时,结石可能会被遮蔽[8]。

十一、膀胱镜检查

膀胱镜检查依然是确诊膀胱结石和选择治疗方案时最常用的检查。这项检查能让术者直视观察结石,测定结石的数量、体积和位置。同时,可对尿道、前列腺、膀胱壁和输尿管口进行检查,对尿道狭窄、前列腺梗阻、膀胱憩室和膀胱肿瘤进行病情评估[8]。

十二、其他检查

盆腔核磁共振(MRI)检查,价格昂贵,对结石分辨率低。因此不推荐 MRI用于膀胱结石的检查诊断。在进行 MRI 检查时,膀胱结石表现为在膀胱腔内出现的低含水量黑洞。与 MRI 一样,锝-99 m、MAG-3 肾扫描也不是进行膀胱结石影像学检查的好方法。但可显示诱发结石的膀胱病灶图像[24]。

十三、组织学检查

长期不接受治疗的膀胱结石可诱使膀胱黏膜异变和诱发膀胱鳞状细胞癌。有时膀胱结石也可附着在移行细胞癌上。膀胱结石成功取出后,留有可疑病灶时,应进行抗感染治疗,并进行活检,以排除可能的恶性病变。

十四、治疗注意事项

膀胱结石本身是一种潜在诱发疾病的临床表现,在去除结石时,这个诱发疾病也应同时得到治疗。治疗诱发结石形成的潜在疾病,如膀胱出口梗阻、感染、异物或饮食等,是预防结石复发的重要部分。治疗膀胱结石的唯一禁忌症是全身状况不佳或晚期无症状的结石患者。

一般情况下,大多数膀胱结石手术都可在内腔镜下实施。然而,如果结石体积太大、质地太硬,或者尿道腔道太细(如儿童或既往尿道手术改变)以致内镜无法插入膀胱时,行耻骨上经膀胱的开放手术则是较好的治疗方法。

十五、药物溶石

药物治疗膀胱结石的目的是溶石、降低死亡率和预防并发症。药物治疗膀胱结石唯一可能有效的方法是碱化尿液,以促使尿酸结石溶解。当尿液 pH 值大于或等于 6.5 时,结石可能被溶解。首选治疗方案是柠檬酸钾(Urocit K)60 mg当量/日。然而,尿液过度碱化后可能会导致磷酸钙沉积在结石表面,进一步对药物治疗失去作用[8]。

其他的溶解结石药物,如 Suby G 溶液或 M 溶液已经很少使用。溶肾石酸素可用于溶解磷酸盐结石,即鸟粪石,但必须要留置导尿管后进行持续冲洗,治疗效果缓慢且对人体有损害,必须严密监控以防患者中毒,即出现高镁血症。为预防结石形成,进一步的措施包括膀胱冲洗、生理盐水机械冲洗碎片或使用上述一种药物治疗方法[21]。

24 h 尿结石疾病分析发现,潜在代谢异常时,应采用相关治疗来防止结石的进一步发展。

参考资料

［1］Douenias R，Rich M，Badlani G，Mazor D，Smith A. Predisposing factors in bladder calculi. Review of 100 cases. Urology. Mar 1991,37(3):240-243.

［2］Hammad F T，Kaya M，Kazim E. Bladder calculi: did the clinical picture change?. Urology. Jun 2006,67(6):1154-1158.

［3］Kamoun A，Daudon M，Abdelmoula J，Hamzaoui M，Chaouachi B，Houissa T，et al. Urolithiasis in Tunisian children: a study of 120 cases based on stone composition. Pediatr Nephrol. Nov 1999,13(9):920-5; discussion 926.

［4］Hodgkinson A. Composition of urinary tract calculi from some developing countries. Urol Int. 1979,34(1):26-35.

［5］Van Reen R. Geographical and nutritional aspects of endemic stones. In: Urinary Calculus. Littleton，Mass: PSG Publishing Co; 1981.

［6］Bakane BC，Nagtilak SB，Patil B. Urolithiasis: a tribal scenario. Indian J Pediatr. Nov-Dec 1999,66(6):863-865.

［7］Bartel P，Krebs J，Wöllner J，Göcking K，Pannek J. Bladder stones in patients with spinal cord injury: a long-term study. Spinal Cord. Apr 2014,52(4):295-297.

［8］Ho K，Segura J. Lower Urinary Tract Calculi. In: Wein A，Kavoussi L，Novick A，Partin A，Peters C. Campbell-Walsh Urology. 3. 9th. Philadelphia，Pa: Saunders Elsevier; 2007:2663-2673.

［9］Ng AC，Leung AK，Robson WL. Urinary bladder calculi in a sliding vesical-inguinal-scrotal hernia diagnosed preoperatively by plain abdominal radiography. Adv Ther. Sep-Oct 2007,24(5):1016-1019.

［10］Mathoera RB，Kok DJ，Nijman RJ. Bladder calculi in augmentation cystoplasty in children. Urology. Sep 1 2000,56(3):482-487.

［11］Rub R，Madeb R，Morgenstern S，Ben-Chaim J，Avidor Y. Development of a large bladder calculus on sutures used for pubic bone closure following extrophy repair. World J Urol. Aug 2001,19(4):261-262.

[12] Godbole P, Mackinnon AE. Expanded PTFE bladder neck slings for incontinence in children: the long-term outcome. BJU Int. Jan 2004,93(1):139-141.

[13] Eichel L, Allende R, Mevorach RA, Hulbert WC, Rabinowitz R. Bladder calculus formation and urinary retention secondary to perforation of a normal bladder by a ventriculoperitoneal shunt. Urology. Aug 2002,60(2):344.

[14] Hick EJ, Hernández J, Yordán R, Morey AF, Avilés R, García CR. Bladder calculus resulting from the migration of an intrauterine contraceptive device. J Urol. Nov 2004, 172(5 Pt 1):1903.

[15] Rafique M. Vesical calculus formation on permanent sutures. J Coll Physicians Surg Pak. Jun 2005,15(6):373-374.

[16] Arunkalaivanan AS, Smith AR. Bladder calculus after laparoscopic colposuspension. J Obstet Gynaecol. Jan 2002,22(1):101.

[17] Lau S, Zammit P, Bikhchandani J, Buchholz NP. The unbreakable bladder stone—Munchhausen's tale. Urol Int. 2006,77(3):284-285.

[18] Russinko PJ, Agarwal S, Choi MJ, Kelty PJ. Obstructive nephropathy secondary to sulfasalazine calculi. Urology. Oct 2003,62(4):748.

[19] Childs MA, Mynderse LA, Rangel LJ, Wilson TM, Lingeman JE, Krambeck AE. Pathogenesis of bladder calculi in the presence of urinary stasis. J Urol. Apr 2013,189 (4):1347-1351.

[20] Mizuno K, Kamisawa H, Hamamoto S, Okamura T, Kohri K. Bilateral single-system ureteroceles with multiple calculi in an adult woman. Urology. Aug 2008, 72 (2):294-295.

[21] Huffman JL, Ginsberg DA. Calculi in the Bladder and Urinary Diversions. In: Coe FL, Favus MJ, Pak CY, Parks JH, Preminger GM, eds. Kidney Stones: Medical and Surgical Management. Philadelphia, Pa: Lippincott-Raven; 1996:1025-1034.

[22] Su CM, Lin HY, Li CC, Chou YH, Huang CH. Bladder stone in a woman after cesarean section: a case report. Kaohsiung J Med Sci. Jan 2003,19(1):42-44.

[23] Huang WC, Yang JM. Sonographic appearance of a bladder calculus secondary to a suture from a bladder neck suspension. J Ultrasound Med. Nov 2002, 21 (11): 1303-1305.

[24] Webb M, Fong W. A large bladder calculus and severe vesicoureteric reflux as seen on

Tc-99 m MAG3 renography. Clin Nucl Med. Nov 2002,27(11):803-804.

（部分内容引自美国 **Medscape** 网站 **Drugs and Diseases** 栏目的 **Bladder Stone** 继续教育内容）

陆鸿海　吴道忻　欧应昌

第二节
膀胱结石的治疗方法

膀胱结石是泌尿外科常见病,目前常用的治疗方法有:①耻骨上膀胱切开取石术;②体外震波碎石术;③经皮耻骨上膀胱穿刺碎石术;④经尿道膀胱碎石术。

一、耻骨上膀胱切开取石术

耻骨上膀胱切开取石术不应作为膀胱结石的首选治疗方法,仅适用于需要同时处理膀胱内其他病变的病例使用。

开放手术的相对适应症:①较复杂的儿童膀胱结石;②巨大膀胱结石;③重度前列腺增生或严重尿道狭窄者;④膀胱憩室内结石;⑤膀胱内围绕异物形成的大结石;⑥同时合并需开放手术的膀胱肿瘤。

在耻骨上膀胱切开取石中,结石不必粉碎可完整取出。该方法可用于大而硬的结石或需要同时行前列腺开放切除术或膀胱憩室切除术的患者,如前列腺大小超过 $80\sim100$ g,考虑行前列腺开放切除术时。

耻骨上膀胱切开取石术的优势包括手术时间短,一次可处理多枚结石。术中更容易取出附着于膀胱黏膜上的结石,可以取出经尿道或经皮膀胱穿刺手术难以击碎或难以取出的大结石和坚硬结石。主要缺点包括手术创伤大、术后切口痛、住院时间和留置尿管时间较长。

二、体外震波碎石术(ESWL)

与肾结石以及大多数输尿管结石不同,大多数医学中心认为,液电碎石和

ESWL 不能有效地治疗膀胱结石[1]。儿童膀胱结石多为原发性结石,可选用 ESWL 治疗。成人≤3 cm 的原发性结石也可以采用 ESWL。但膀胱结石多坚硬,而膀胱空腔大,碎石时,结石容易在膀胱腔内滚动,碎石效率低。一些研究提示,可采用俯卧位进行 ESWL,碎石效果较好[2]。因此在美国,有些医院应用 ESWL 治疗膀胱结石时,通常会采用俯卧位进行碎石。

三、经皮耻骨上膀胱穿刺碎石术

近年来,对于 2 cm 以上的大体积膀胱结石,国外多有报道采用经皮耻骨上膀胱穿刺插入镜鞘,再通过镜鞘插入肾镜或膀胱镜,应用钬激光或气压弹道进行碎石,疗效较好。在经皮耻骨上膀胱穿刺碎石术中,可允许采用长度较短和直径较大的内窥镜插入膀胱,再使用超声波碎石机等设备,从而能加快碎石和取石的速度。目前,经皮膀胱穿刺碎石方法通常是治疗小儿膀胱结石的首选途径[3]。

Paez 等报道,在一项研究中,在超声引导下行耻骨上膀胱穿刺建立手术通道,再实施经皮膀胱碎石术,未发现手术有特殊并发症发生,故认为经皮耻骨上膀胱穿刺碎石术是一种安全、可选择的手术方法。与这种相同的治疗方法也有报道应用于尿道闭锁或尿流改道的患者[4]。但是对于>4 cm 的膀胱结石,这种方法的疗效明显下降,建议采用耻骨上膀胱切开取石术。

四、经尿道膀胱碎石术

经尿道膀胱碎石术是在摄像视屏监控下,内镜经过尿道进入膀胱,直视下寻及膀胱结石后,应用碎石设备击碎结石,再通过内镜取出碎石的手术方法。碎石设备可以是物理碎石设备,即气压弹道碎石、超声波碎石、液电碎石、激光碎石,也可以是手工碎石器械。由于是利用尿道这一人体自然通道进入膀胱进行碎石,因此对人体损伤较小。近年来膀胱结石的治疗方法得到不断改进,经尿道膀胱碎石已成为最主要的手术方法。随着医疗器械的不断改进,已经能够通过儿童较小口径的尿道,因此该方法现在也适用于合适的儿童[5]。

1. 经尿道机械碎石术

经尿道机械碎石术采用膀胱碎石镜,利用机械力学原理,通过碎石钳咬合力的机械挤压将结石粉碎。术中,在膀胱碎石镜直视下用碎石钳将结石抓住,并用机械力将结石钳碎。适用于 2 cm 以下的膀胱结石。由于膀胱碎石镜在插入膀胱,粉碎结石,取出碎石的过程中容易损伤膀胱、尿道黏膜,故临床上已很少使用。

2. 经尿道钬激光碎石术

经尿道钬激光碎石术是利用现有的内镜设备,如膀胱镜、输尿管镜、肾镜或电切镜等作为碎石平台,采用钬激光光纤,通过上述内镜平台经尿道粉碎膀胱结石。结石粉碎后再用配套的异物钳、电切镜配套的电切襻,摄取碎石或用冲洗器冲取碎石。钬激光碎石通常速度较缓慢,即使用 1 000 μm 的光纤也是这样[6]。但是对极大部分结石均有效,可用于治疗不同成分和结构的膀胱结石,在国内已经成为膀胱结石的主要治疗方法。

3. 经尿道气压弹道碎石术

经尿道气压弹道碎石术是采用气压弹道碎石杆,通过内镜碎石平台经尿道治疗膀胱结石。气压弹道碎石也是目前常用的一种有效的碎石方法。

4. 经尿道超声碎石术

经尿道超声碎石术用于经尿道膀胱碎石,目前已经较少使用。

1963 年,Baranes 等首先描述并被大量文献所支持,认为经尿道碎石术联合经尿道前列腺切除术(TURP)或经尿道前列腺切开术(TUIP)可以顺利完成,并且是安全的[7, 8]。建议术中先处理结石再治疗前列腺;反之,则可能出现出血、液体过度吸收等并发症。Tugcu 等报道对 64 例 TURP 术患者同时实施膀胱结石手术[9]。这些患者采用两种碎石治疗方法：①取 F30 镜鞘经皮耻骨上途径穿刺插入膀胱；②F23 镜鞘经尿道膀胱碎石术，均采用气压弹道碎石。经皮碎石患者的结石负荷更大，具有统计学差异。经皮途径碎石的平均手术时间仅是经尿道碎石患者的一半左右。因此膀胱结石过大、过多时，也可采用经尿道途径联合经皮耻骨上途径，用来帮助固定结石和方便碎石的冲洗。

五、现有内镜设备用于膀胱碎石时的不足

使用膀胱镜、输尿管镜、肾镜或电切镜等现有内镜设备作为经尿道碎石平台，具有手术时无法克服的关键性和共性的技术难题：

（1）由于膀胱空腔大，结石容易在腔内滑动，因此膀胱结石不易粉碎，碎石效率不高。

（2）碎石时，结石在膀胱腔内跳动，撞击膀胱壁，易引起黏膜损伤出血。

（3）结石滑动后或破裂时，钬激光易损伤膀胱黏膜。

（4）在治疗多发性膀胱结石，或大体积膀胱结石粉碎后形成大量碎石时，现有异物钳或电切襻等设备不易快速取出碎石。尤其是男性患者，由于尿道弯曲而细长更不易去除。

（5）膀胱壁充盈后变薄，容易损伤穿孔。

现有的膀胱镜、输尿管镜、肾镜或电切镜等内镜可用于治疗膀胱结石，为碎石设备提供碎石操作平台，但效率不能令人满意。同时，结石粉碎后缺乏理想的取石方法将碎石快速取净。各种内镜配套的异物钳和电切镜配套的电切襻可用于术中摄取碎石，但结构设计上存在缺陷，容易造成损耗。功能上只能摄取体积较小的碎石，不能固定结石。因此，目前由于缺乏理想的手术器械，现有内镜设备仅适用于经尿道治疗直径小于 2～3 cm 的膀胱结石。

参考资料

[1] Losty P, Surana R, O'Donnell B. Limitations of extracorporeal shock wave lithotripsy for urinary tract calculi in young children. J Pediatr Surg. Aug 1993, 28（8）: 1037-1039.

[2] Bhatia V, Biyani CS. Vesical lithiasis: open surgery versus cystolithotripsy versus ex-

tracorporeal shock wave therapy. J Urol. Mar 1994,151(3):660-662.

[3] Ikari O，Netto NR Jr，D'Ancona CA，Palma PC. Percutaneous treatment of bladder stones. J Urol. Jun 1993,149(6):1499-1500.

[4] Franzoni DF，Decter RM. Percutaneous vesicolithotomy：an alternative to open bladder surgery in patients with an impassable or surgically ablated urethra. J Urol. Sep 1999, 162(3 Pt 1):777-778.

[5] Shokeir AA. Transurethral cystolitholapaxy in children. J Endourol. Apr 1994,8(2): 157-159; discussion 159-160.

[6] Wollin TA，Singal RK，Whelan T，Dicecco R，Razvi HA，Denstedt JD. Percutaneous suprapubic cystolithotripsy for treatment of large bladder calculi. J Endourol. Dec 1999,13(10):739-744.

[7] Barnes RW，Bergman RT，Worton E. Litholapaxy vs. cystolithotomy. J Urol. May 1963,89:680-681.

[8] Nseyo UO，Rivard DJ，Garlick WB，Bennett AH. Management of bladder stones： should transurethral prostatic resection be performed in combination with cystolitholapaxy?. Urology. Mar 1987,29(3):265-267.

[9] Tugcu V，Polat H，Ozbay B，Gurbuz N，Eren GA，Tasci AI. Percutaneous versus transurethral cystolithotripsy. J Endourol. Feb 2009,23(2):237-241.

（部分内容引自美国 Medscape 网站 Drugs and Diseases 栏目的 Bladder Stone 继续教育内容）

李威武　方　炜　朱仙华

AH-1 型取石系统的技术方案、实验数据和临床用途

采用现有的内镜碎石技术治疗膀胱结石时,结石无法固定,容易在膀胱内滑动,碎石效率不高,易损伤出血;结石粉碎后缺乏快速有效的手段清除碎石,这些问题严重影响了腔内微创手术治疗膀胱结石的效率。因此,临床上需要一种能将膀胱结石固定后再进行碎石,结石粉碎后又能快速、高效地清除碎石的多功能内镜。为了解决上述不足,结合现有的各种内镜、异物钳和碎石设备的技术特点,我们研制了 AH-1 型取石系统(图 3-1、图 3-2)。为临床医生提供了一种集合检查诊断、固定结石、提供碎石通道、摄取碎石、冲吸碎石和可连续冲洗等功能为一体的多功能内镜。

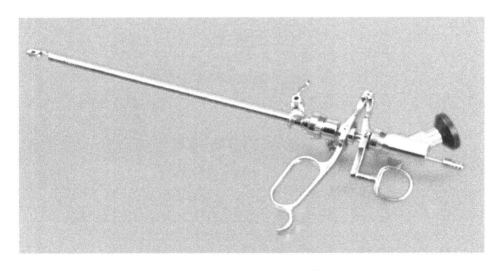

图 3-1　AH-1 型取石系统

一、技术方案

AH-1 型取石系统由以下八个部分组成。

1. 镜鞘

镜鞘附有内芯(闭孔器),入镜时置入内芯或镜桥,入镜后用于连接镜体,进行下一步操作。镜鞘也可连接冲吸器,冲吸碎石。

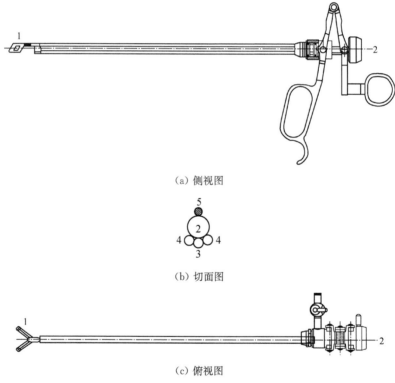

(a) 侧视图

(b) 切面图

(c) 俯视图

图 3-2 AH-1 型取石系统总装图

1—取石钳;2—窥镜插入通道;3—碎石通道;4—进水通道;5—取石钳拉杆通道

2. 液体连续冲洗系统

镜体上缘设有进水通道管,连接进水阀。镜体和镜鞘的间隙为出水通道,与出水阀相连接。用于术中持续冲洗,保持视野清晰。

3. 插入式窥镜

插入式窥镜(图 3-3),包含窥镜光源、成像系统。用于术中的成像、定位。

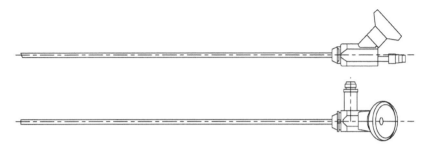

图 3-3　插入式窥镜

4. 取石钳

取石钳由钳夹和拉杆组成,用于固定结石、摄取碎石。钳夹固定于镜体前端上缘,钳片向下,通过拉杆与手柄相连。手柄在镜体滑槽中移动后牵动拉杆,拉杆再拉动钳片,使钳夹产生开启和闭合运动,抓持物体。纵视钳片弯曲呈弧形,钳夹为环状,有利于抓持、摄取结石时的视野观察。钳片顶端内缘设有阻挡襻,可在镜鞘内进行拉网状一次抓取多枚结石。取石钳片如图 3-4 所示。

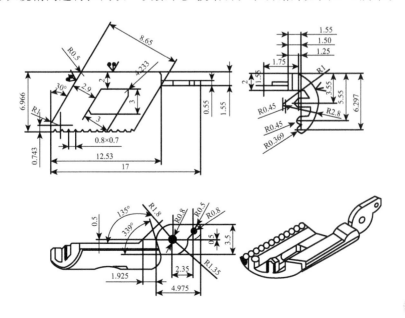

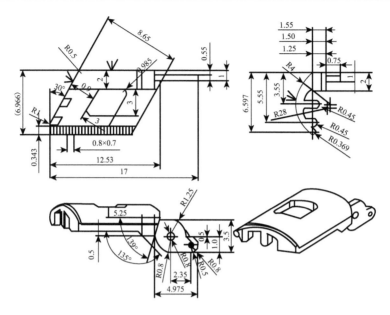

图 3-4　左右取石钳片(固定于镜体前部上缘,钳片向下)

5. 碎石通道

碎石器械的操作通道,可通过气压弹道碎石杆和激光碎石光纤进行碎石操作。扩大碎石通道后,也可应用 EMS 碎石机进行碎石操作。

6. 镜桥

镜桥内插入窥镜后再插入镜鞘,与普通膀胱尿道镜相似,直视下经尿道进入膀胱,进行相关的膀胱、尿道检查和其他操作,如图 3-5 所示。

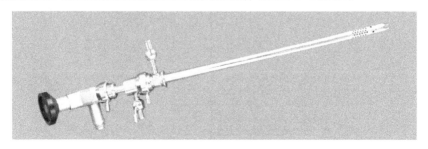

图 3-5　与镜鞘相连并已插入窥镜的镜桥

7．多用途镜鞘连接转换器

通过镜鞘连接转换器,可将 AH-1 型取石系统与各种型号的电切镜外鞘进行连接,增强 AH-1 型取石系统的通用性。

8．冲吸器

冲吸器可与镜鞘连接,冲吸细小碎石。

二、镜体横截剖面结构分布

（1）如图 3-6 所示,镜体横截剖面上排是取石钳拉杆通道,中间是窥镜通道,下排是碎石通道,其两侧为冲水通道。

（2）窥镜光源、成像系统置于镜体横截剖面的中间通道,便于视野观察。同时窥镜可获得有效保护,不易损坏。

（3）取石钳拉杆位于镜体上排通道,钳夹位于物镜前端上缘,由钳片由上向下开启,便于观察和抓持、固定、摄取结石。

（4）碎石操作通道位于横截剖面的下排,物镜和光源的下缘,便于直视下抓取结石和碎石操作。

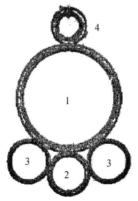

图 3-6　镜体横截剖面结构分布

1—窥镜通道;2—碎石光纤通道;3—进水通道;4—取石钳拉杆通道

三、体外实验数据

为了安全、有效地将 AH-1 型取石系统应用于临床治疗膀胱结石,在临床应用前进行了体外实验,临床应用中可参考和应用这些实验数据,如图 3-7 所示。

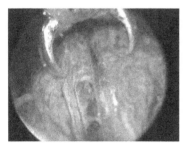 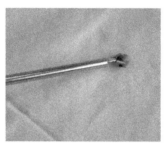 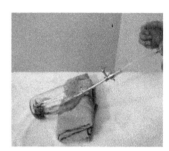

(a) 钳夹固定冲击实验　　　　　(b) 钳夹摄取实验　　　　　(c) 冲吸实验

图 3-7　体外实验

1. 实验设备

(1) F26 AH-1 型取石系统,由杭州时空候医疗器械有限公司生产。

(2) 德国产 Wolf 气压弹道碎石机,碎石杆直径 1.2 mm。

2. 实验材料

(1) 胡桃,直径 28 mm;

(2) 冲吸气囊,直径 60 mm;

(3) 大西米,直径 5.7 mm;

(4) 黄豆,直径 8.2 mm;

(5) 莲芯,直径 13 mm;

(6) 花生,直径 15 mm;

(7) 赤豆,直径 6.3 mm。

3. 实验目的

体外实验试图通过对 AH-1 型取石系统样件的设计构件进行实物测定,并对不同直径的圆球体进行体外实物测试,以检验 AH-1 型取石系统设计功能的实际有效性。

4. 实验结论

(1) 固定结石功能

AH-1 型取石系统取石钳片长 12 mm,两侧钳片外展 70°,钳夹合计外展可达 140°。在气压弹道碎石杆的冲击下,利用钳夹的咬合力和向下压力,可有效固定直径 60 mm 的球体,因此理论上可固定无限大结石,达到碎石操作时具有固定结石功能的设计要求。

(2) 摄取结石功能

① 鞘内摄取结石:镜鞘最大内径 8.2 mm,取石钳夹闭合后最小内径 4 mm。应用钳夹,可在镜鞘内顺利摄取直径小于 8 mm 球体。

② 带鞘摄取结石:在镜鞘外可摄取最大圆球体直径 15 mm。

(3) 碎石通道功能

碎石通道内径 1.4 mm,可通过目前最大的 500 μm 钬激光光纤和小于 1.4 mm 的气压弹道碎石杆,进行碎石操作。

(4) 冲吸结石功能

镜鞘镜鞘外径 F26(8.7 mm),内径 F25(8.3 mm)。通过最大圆球体的直径 8.2 mm。测试冲吸直径 6.3 mm 球体时效率良好。

(5) 连续冲洗流量

两根进水通道内径 1.4 mm,出水通道为镜鞘和镜体的空隙,横截面较大。公式为

$$Q = S \cdot V = \prod R^2 \cdot \sqrt{2HG}$$

式中　Q——流量;

　　　S——管道截面积;

　　　V——水在管道内流速;

$\prod$—— 3.14;

H—— 高度;

G—— 比重。

在设定冲洗液容器与镜体垂直高度为100 mm时,理论流量为 409 ml/min。实际测得进水流量为 200 ml/min。

四、临床用途和功能

(1) 经尿道进行膀胱检查诊断。

(2) 固定结石,便于碎石操作,提高碎石效率。

(3) 配用气压弹道碎石、激光碎石设备进行碎石操作。

(4) 回旋流自动收集碎石,其原理如图 3-8 所示。

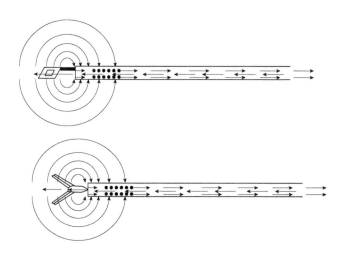

图 3-8　回旋流自动收集碎石原理

(5) 镜鞘内拉网状一次摄取多枚碎石。

(6) 连接冲洗器后冲吸碎石。

(7) 术中液体连续冲洗。

(8) 用于摄取各种其他膀胱异物。

(9) 通过镜鞘连接转换器可与各种型号的电切镜外鞘连接。

(10) 直径减小后用于经皮肾盂结石的碎石操作。

（11）前列腺剜除术中切割、摄取已剜除的前列腺组织。

（12）研制中 F22 的 AH-2 型取石系统直径缩小。将用于经皮肾结石碎石手术，可替代肾镜功能的同时加速摄取肾盂碎石的操作。

（13）直径减小后的 AH-2 型取石系统可用于治疗小儿膀胱结石。

五、临床实施方式

采用 AH-1 型取石系统治疗膀胱结石时，先将内芯置入镜鞘内，然后经尿道将镜鞘插入膀胱，或更换镜桥后直视下将镜鞘插入膀胱；入镜后将镜体置入镜鞘内，也可通过镜鞘连接转换器与已经置入膀胱的电切镜外鞘连接；检查、寻找结石；寻及结石后再用取石钳的咬合，下压力固定结石；然后将气压弹道碎石杆或激光碎石光纤通过碎石通道进行碎石；结石粉碎后利用回旋流自动收集碎石，同时应用取石钳夹在镜鞘内拉网状抓取碎石，有大量细小碎石时，镜鞘可连接冲吸器，冲吸碎石。

李爱华　张　晔　王　绮

第四节
AH-1 型取石系统经尿道膀胱
碎石术的规范化方案

一、治疗膀胱结石的目的和原则

（1）取出结石；

（2）纠正形成结石的原因。

二、手术适应证

绝大多数无严重尿道狭窄的膀胱结石都可采用 AH-1 型取石系统经尿道治疗,目前已经治疗的最大结石直径为 6.6 cm。结石的直径每增加 1 cm,手术难度将增加 1 倍,随着结石体积的增大、数量的增多,相应的碎石时间和取石时间也会延长。对于结石体积过大、数目过多的高危、高龄患者,可分期进行手术。

伴有前列腺增生时可同时实施 TURP 术。建议先行碎石,再行 TURP 术。尿道狭窄者一般需要在尿道扩张后再实施碎石手术。

三、术前准备

（1）KUB,KUB＋IVP,B 超或 CT 等影像学检查,明确结石大小和数目,查明诱发结石的原因。

（2）尿常规检查及尿细菌培养，了解有无尿路感染，如有合并感染应先控制感染，如果有难以控制的反复感染，可在敏感抗生素保护下手术。

（3）如有造成尿液反流引起肾积水的梗阻，可先引流尿液，改善肾功能。

（4）合并严重内科疾病的膀胱结石患者，可先行导尿或耻骨上膀胱穿刺造瘘。待内科疾病好转，麻醉评分允许后再实施碎石手术。

四、麻醉和体位

一般采用腰麻或硬膜外麻醉，如有腰椎病变可改用全麻。手术体位均采用膀胱截石位。

五、手术步骤

（1）对尿道狭小者常规行尿道扩张。

（2）先将内芯（闭孔器）置入镜鞘内，然后经尿道将镜鞘插入膀胱。

（3）因尿道狭小，进一步插入困难时拔出内芯，置入镜桥，直视下将镜鞘插入膀胱。

（4）入镜后将镜体置入镜鞘内，常规全面检查膀胱，寻找结石。

（5）寻及结石后，应用取石钳咬合、下压，以固定结石。

（6）将气压弹道碎石杆或激光碎石光纤通过碎石通道插入膀胱，进行碎石操作。

（7）结石粉碎后，在连续冲洗下利用回旋流自动收集碎石，同时应用取石钳夹在镜鞘内拉网状摄取碎石。

（8）残留大量细小碎石时，可将冲吸器连接镜鞘，冲吸碎石。

（9）对伴有前列腺增生的患者，结石取净后再按常规行 TURP 术。

（10）钬激光碎石功率一般设定在 $30\sim60$ W 之间。

六、手术并发症及处理

1. 膀胱穿孔

采用 AH-1 型取石系统经尿道膀胱钬激光碎石或气压弹道碎石是一种轻度侵袭性的治疗方法,目前尚无膀胱损伤导致膀胱穿孔的病例。但同样具有潜在并发症发生的可能。如有大的膀胱穿孔时,应立即中止操作,转开放手术,行膀胱裂口修补术。

2. 血尿

碎石过程中尿道和膀胱黏膜损伤小、出血少,一般无需特殊处理。严重时,可留置三腔导尿管,持续膀胱冲洗。同时施行 TURP 时,应按 TURP 术的操作程序处理血尿。

七、术后处理

(1) 术后常规留置导尿。

(2) 多饮水,适当抗生素治疗。

(3) 单纯膀胱结石患者术后 48 h 拔除尿管。

(4) 同时行 TURP 时按 TURP 术处理,术后 5～7 天拔除尿管。

(5) 术后 3～4 周进行 KUB 摄片或膀胱超声检查,以评估残留碎石的排除情况。

(6) 随后每 6～12 月 KUB 摄片检查一次。

(7) 尿酸结石、伴有上尿路结石、有明显结石家族史、无尿路梗阻和复发性结石的患者应进行结石成分的代谢分析。

八、碎石设备的选择

1. 钬激光碎石机

选用功率在 30 W 以上的钬激光碎石机。碎石通道可通过较粗的碎石光纤，一般选用 500 μm 的光纤。

2. 气压弹道碎石机

选用合适直径的碎石杆。输尿管镜用的碎石杆用于 AH-1 型取石系统时由于长度过长，故无法使用。术前可用口腔科的切割工具预先切除碎石杆的过长部分，使碎石杆的长短适用于 AH-1 型取石系统。

九、操作体会

（1）为避免意外损伤，镜鞘置入膀胱后应直视下插入带有取石钳的操作件。

（2）尿道狭窄时，应先行尿道扩张，镜鞘插入尿道后拔出内芯，再插入镜桥。直视下将镜鞘插入膀胱，减少对尿道黏膜的损伤。

（3）前列腺中叶过大、颈部过高，使碎石操作无法进行，或前列腺体积过大阻塞后尿道使镜鞘无法插入膀胱时，可先行 TURP 切除抬高的膀胱颈部或过大的前列腺，以便镜鞘能顺利插入膀胱。此时应加强手术创面的止血，减少创面渗血，避免影响下一步的手术操作。

（4）较大的结石可以在镜鞘外直接取出，但这样的操作对尿道黏膜损伤大，不宜反复使用。

（5）术中使用低压持续冲洗，可保持视野清晰，避免膀胱黏膜损伤。

（6）正常情况下，宜先碎石再行 TURP。这样的操作顺序可避免 TURP 术后手术创面的渗血而影响手术视野，以及过多吸收冲洗液。

（7）对于高龄高危、结石体积过大或数目过多的患者，可采用分期碎石的治疗方案。

（8）碎石时，注意击打结石的要害部分，可利用取石钳和激光光纤或碎石杆转动结石，移动结石的位置，调节结石的击打部位。

（9）摄取碎石时，注意取石钳和镜鞘之间的配合，避免夹住膀胱黏膜，造成意外损伤。

（10）体积大的结石可在碎石的同时分批摄取碎石，体积小的结石可一次粉碎后再摄取碎石。

（11）粉碎低比重的结石时会出现结石上浮，在膀胱腔内四处浮动的现象，给碎石操作带来巨大困难。此时应设法抓住结石，将结石下压后再碎石。

（12）对于膀胱容量小的大体积结石，有时膀胱容量过小，导致工作空间过小取石钳无法插入。此时结石在膀胱内较固定，不易滑动，可不必坚持先插入取石钳再碎石，避免强行插入造成意外损伤取石钳。可先换用其他内镜作为碎石平台进行碎石，待结石部分粉碎，膀胱空间加大后再换用取石钳固定碎石，抓取碎石。

张　峰　李进红　吴文美

AH-1 型取石系统经尿道膀胱碎石疗效与现有方法的比较评估

[摘要] **目的:**评估 AH-1 型取石系统(SRS 系统)治疗膀胱结石的安全性和疗效。**方法:**采用 SRS 系统经尿道碎石+经尿道前列腺电切术(TURP)治疗的膀胱结石伴前列腺增生(BPH)74 例结石患者,与经尿道输尿管镜碎石+TURP 治疗的 50 例结石患者的临床资料进行回顾性比较。对直径<2 cm 和≥2 cm 结石分别评估。**结果:**SRS 组<2 cm 结石和≥2 cm 结石患者的结石直径均大于对照组,<2 cm 结石的差异有统计学意义,$P<0.001$。两组相比,<2 cm 结石患者的总手术时间和结石清除时间差异有统计学意义($P<0.02$, $P<0.001$)。单发性≥2 cm 结石患者的总手术时间和结石清除时间差异有显著性,$P<0.05$。≥2 cm 结石组清除一枚结石所需平均手术时间差异有统计学意义,$P<0.001$。SRS 系统组无严重并发症发生。**结论:**SRS 系统可提供固定结石、提供碎石通道、自动收集碎石、摄取碎石、冲吸碎石和连续冲洗等功能。尤其是可固定结石、自动收集碎石、一次可摄取多枚碎石。可缩短手术时间,拓展内镜治疗膀胱结石的手术适应范围。其联合 TURP 用于治疗膀胱结石伴 BPH 是一种安全、有效的治疗方法。

[关键词] 膀胱结石;经尿道碎石;内镜;AH-1 型取石系统

The Efficiency of Transurethral Cystolithotripsy with AH-1 Stone Removal System Compared with Current Methods

ABSTRACT　Objective： To evaluate the safety and efficiency of Aihua (AH)-1 stone removal system(SRS) to treat bladder stone. **Methods：** Seventy four patients with bladder stone and benign prostatic hyperplasia(BPH) were treated by transurethral cystolithotripsy with SRS and TURP. The results in these patients were compared with 50 patients treated with current devices. Patients with stone$<$2 cm and $\geqslant$2 cm were respectively compared between the two groups. **Results：** SRS group was compared with control group，the difference of stone size in patients with stone $<$2 cm was statistically significant，$P<0.001$. The difference of total operating time，$P<0.02$ and stone removal time，$P<0.001$ was statistically significant in patients with stone $<$2 cm. The difference of total operating time and stone removal time was statistically significant in patients with single stone $\geqslant$2 cm，$P<0.05$. The difference of mean time to remove one stone was statistically significant in patients with stone $\geqslant$2 cm，$P<0.001$. No significant complication was found in SRS group. **Conclusion：** This study suggests that multiple functions of SRS can be expected in transurethral cystolithotripsy. It can be used to fix stones during lithotripsy，and automatically collect stones and extract more stones through the sheath at one time during lithoextraction，which can reduce surgical time and damage to the bladder and urethra. This surgical procedure appears to be safe and efficient，and operating indications for transurethral cystolithotripsy could be expanded with this surgical procedure.

Key words　Bladder stone；Transurethral Cystolithotripsy；Endoscope；AH-1 Stone Removal System

近十年来膀胱结石的治疗方法得到不断改进,经尿道碎石已经成为最主要的方法[1-9]。但是目前不同的经尿道膀胱碎石术依然存在一些重大缺陷,术中无法固定结石、不能进行持续冲洗、碎石取出较困难,当结石直径大于 2 cm 时,手术难度将明显增加。为了解决上述缺陷，我们研制了 AH-1 型取石系统（Aihua-1 Stone removal System，SRS），其具有固定结石、提供碎石通道、自动收集碎石、冲吸碎石、摄取碎石和连续冲洗等功能[10-11]。SRS 系统由李爱华发明设计，杭州时空候医疗器械有限公司生产。本文对照常用的输尿管镜联合电切镜膀胱碎石术，回顾性探讨 SRS 系统治疗膀胱结石的安全性和疗效，现报告如下。

一、材料与方法

1. 临床资料

我院 2008 年 1 月至 2012 年 12 月年共采用 SRS 系统联合 TURP 一期治疗治疗膀胱结石伴前列腺增生（Benign Prostatic Hyperplasia，BPH）74 例，患者平均年龄 74.3 岁。对照组输尿管镜碎石联合经尿道前列腺电切术（Trans Urethral Resection Prostate，TURP）治疗膀胱结石伴 BPH 50 例，患者平均年龄 73.2 岁。分别对直径＜2 cm 和≥2 cm 结石进行评估，统计结石数目时包含所有≥1 cm 结石。

2. 手术器械和方法

各组均在脊柱麻醉下取截石位，钬激光碎石所用功率为 2.6～3.5 J 和 2.0～2.5 Hz。

SRS 组[10-11] F26 SRS 系统由窥镜光源成像系统、手柄、取石钳、碎石通道、液体连续冲洗系统、镜桥、镜鞘等部件组成（图 5-1）。可用取石钳钳夹固定直径＞6 cm 的球体。镜鞘内径 8.2 mm，可与 Ellick 冲吸器连接。镜鞘内可摄取直径＜0.8 cm 的球体，镜鞘外可摄取直径＜1.5 cm 的球体。碎石通道内径 1.4 mm，可通过气压弹道碎石杆或钬激光光纤。术中可通过镜桥直视下经尿道置入 SRS 系统，然后更换取石钳，寻及结石后固定结石。应用钬激光粉碎结石，再用取石钳或 Ellick 冲吸器取出碎石，然后行 TURP。

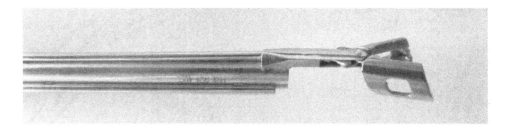

图 5-1　取石钳实物图

对照组[3]经尿道置入 F26 连续冲洗型 Storze 电切镜,寻及结石后用镜鞘固定。镜鞘内置入 F8 Storze 输尿管镜,钬激光碎石后再行 TURP。

3. 统计学方法

对数据资料均以均数±标准误表示,采用两独立样本的 t 检验进行差异显著性检验。假设检验的显著性水平取 $\alpha=0.05$。

二、结果

1. 患者基本临床资料

两组患者的临床基本资料见表 5-1。

表 5-1　患者临床资料

项目	病例 N	年龄/岁	结石直径/cm	前列腺体积/ml
		<2 cm 结石		
SRS组	30	70.66±10.19	1.39±0.31	42.09±23.63
对照组	36	70.26±10.13	0.98±0.40	51.18±27.81
t 值		1.025 6	4.562 6	1.113 8
P 值		>0.05	<0.001	>0.05

(续表)

项目	病例 N	年龄/岁	结石直径/cm	前列腺体积/ml
		≥2 cm 结石		
SRS组	44	76.48±8.76	3.11±1.06	56.44±38.20
对照组	14	74.07±12.88	2.54±0.46	52.16±43.80
t 值		0.795 2	1.947 7	0.320 8
P 值		>0.05	>0.05	>0.05

SRS组<2 cm 和≥2 cm 结石的直径均大于对照组,<2 cm 结石的差异有统计学意义($P<0.001$),两组间年龄和前列腺体积差异无统计学意义。

2. 手术疗效

两组患者的手术情况见表 5-2 和表 5-3。

表 5-2 直径<2 cm 和单发性≥2 cm 结石患者的手术时间

项目	病例 N	结石直径/cm	总手术时间/min	碎石时间/min
		<2 cm 结石		
SRS组	30	1.39±0.31	46.81±15.00	8.83±10.58
对照组	36	0.98±0.40	62.51±25.43	28.95±27.49
t 值		4.562 6	2.513 9	3.719 7
P 值		<0.001	<0.02	<0.001
项目		单发≥2 cm 结石		
SRS组	30	3.21±1.02	54.07±19.57	21.93±16.72
对照组	12	2.46±0.45	79.85±24.63	43.28±24.18
t 值		0.486 5	3.531 2	3.251 9
P 值		>0.05	<0.01	<0.01

表 5-3 清除一枚直径≥2 cm 结石所需平均手术时间

项目	SRS组	对照组	t 值	P 值
病例 N	44	14		
累计结石数目	81	17		
平均结石数目	1.84±1.88	1.21±0.43	1.237 0	>0.05
结石直径/cm	2.48±1.07	2.45±0.47	0.300 0	>0.05
平均手术时间/min	12.84±14.04	33.23±25.26	4.650 6	<0.001

两组相比,直径<2 cm结石的总手术时间和结石清除时间差异有统计学意义($P<0.02$,$P<0.001$)。单发性直径≥2 cm结石的总手术时间和结石清除时间差异有显著性($P<0.01$)。

在直径<2 cm结石中,SRS组15例(50.00%)为多发性结石,对照组为23例(63.89%)。直径≥2 cm结石中,SRS组14例(31.82%)为多发性结石,对照组为2例(14.29%)。

两组相比,清除一枚结石所需平均手术时间差异有统计学意义($P<0.001$)。

SRS组<2 cm结石患者的结石直径较大,其中4例直接用取石钳取出,其余26例为碎石后取出。对照组<2 cm结石中4例直接用Ellick冲吸器取出,15例用电切襻取出,其余16例为碎石后取出。≥2 cm结石均需碎石后才能取出。

3. 手术并发症比较

对照组术中转开放手术3例(6.00%)。一例为直径3.2 cm结石,结构坚硬,无法用镜鞘固定,碎石时结石在膀胱腔内不断滑动,钬激光碎石效率无法发挥。改用输尿管镜直接碎石,由于不能持续冲洗,手术视野模糊。手术进行1 h后发现膀胱黏膜损伤导致膀胱壁破裂。两例由于碎石过多无法取净,3个月后继发尿道狭窄。

SRS组无特殊并发症发生,无中转开放手术。一例为97岁多发性结石患者,其中最大结石直径5.8 cm,一枚结石直径2.2 cm,其余15枚结石小于2 cm,为手术安全碎石102 min后终止手术,2周后再行碎石。另有四例患者伴有尿道狭窄或尿道内径过小,先行尿道扩张,改用F24电切镜行TURP,然后碎石。此时,由于前列腺窝创面渗血,手术视野较模糊。

三、讨论

现有腔内微创技术仅适用于直径小于2 cm的膀胱结石[12],其主要原因是术中常遇的以下六大难题:①膀胱空腔大,膀胱结石多大而坚硬,碎石时容易在腔内滑动;②碎石时结石在膀胱腔内跳动,撞击膀胱壁易引起黏膜损伤出血;③结石滑动后钬激光易损伤膀胱黏膜;④结石粉碎后形成大量碎石,加之尿道弯曲,现有设备不易取出;⑤膀胱壁充盈后变薄,容易损伤穿孔;⑥部分内镜无法连续冲洗,导致视野不清。

应用输尿管镜联合电切镜进行膀胱碎石是一种有效的方法[3],但是镜鞘固定结石的稳定性远不如SRS系统的取石钳,结石过大时常无法固定结石。碎石时,结石经常在膀胱腔内不断滑动,钬激光碎石效率无法有效发挥。用输尿管镜直接碎石,由于输尿管镜进水流量小,又不能持续冲洗,手术视野常模糊不清,容易损伤膀胱黏膜。一旦黏膜损伤出血,视野将更加模糊。加之膀胱壁充盈后变薄,容易损伤穿孔。因此在处理较大结石时容易损伤膀胱黏膜导致膀胱壁破裂。术中,细小结石可采用Ellick冲吸器冲吸,也可用电切襻在操作腔内或镜鞘外取出较大碎石,但取石效率低,容易损坏电切襻。反复使用后容易损坏电切镜上用于锁定电切襻的固定器。本文两例由于碎石后产生过多碎石,无法彻底取净,最终改行开放手术。其次,经尿道反复插入电切镜取石会严重损伤尿道黏膜,可导致术后继发性尿道狭窄发生。因此该方法更适用于直径小于2 cm的结石。

SRS系统是一种金属硬性内镜。取石钳位于物镜的前端,由上向下张合,钳夹闭合时纵观呈圆形,其中央部依然为圆形腔道(图5-2)。取石钳夹片呈框架状,碎石时易于抓取、固定结石。钳夹的顶端边缘设有阻挡襻,可在镜鞘内进行拖网式取石,一次可取出多枚结石。金属钳夹可有力地控制6.4 cm以下的结石,进行碎石操作。镜鞘也可

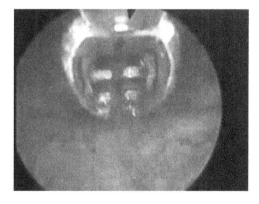

图5-2 内镜下的取石钳

与冲吸器相连,冲吸结石。应用流体力学回旋流原理,带有出水孔的镜鞘使SRS系统具有自动收集结石的功能。碎石通道位于物镜和光源的下缘,便于在直视下抓取结石,进行碎石操作。

术中,SRS系统可在直视下入镜,结石固定后再进行碎石操作,此时,结石无法在膀胱腔内滑动,用钬激光或气压弹道碎石时碎石效率大幅提高,结石容

易粉碎(图5-3)。其次,SRS系统具有连续冲洗功能,进、出水流量大,术中可保持清晰视野,便于操作,不易损伤膀胱黏膜。结石粉碎后,用SRS系统的取石钳在镜鞘内拖网式取石,一次可取出多枚碎石(图5-4)。有较多细小碎石时也可采用冲吸器冲吸取石。同时,SRS系统的镜鞘内径远大于F26连续冲洗型Storze电切镜的操作内径,可取出更大碎石,可明显提高取石效率,缩短手术时间。不同于电切镜的电切襻取石方法,SRS系统的取石钳取石操作一般都是在镜鞘内进行,可有效减少镜鞘反复插入尿道导致的尿道黏膜损伤。

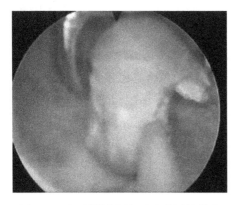 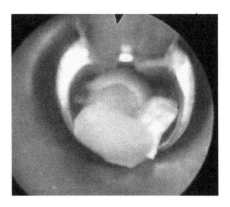

图5-3　取石钳固定结石后采用钬激光　　图5-4　取石钳在镜鞘内一次抓取出
　　　　进行碎石　　　　　　　　　　　　　　　多枚碎石

　　为避免意外损伤,SRS系统镜鞘置入膀胱后应直视下插入取石钳。如结石较大,可在镜鞘外直接取出,但这样的操作对尿道黏膜损伤大,不宜反复使用。术中保持低压持续冲洗,可保持视野清晰,避免膀胱黏膜损伤。推荐碎石后再行TURP,这样更易操作。对于高龄、高危、结石体积过大和数目过多的患者,可采用分期碎石治疗。

　　总之,SRS系统是一种集固定结石、提供碎石通道、自动收集碎石、摄取碎石、冲吸碎石和连续冲洗等功能为一体的多功能内镜。尤其是术中可固定结石、自动收集碎石、一次可摄取多枚碎石。与现有方法比较,可缩短手术时间,提高碎石效率,减少意外损伤,拓展内镜治疗膀胱结石的手术适应范围。其联合TURP用于治疗膀胱结石伴BPH,是一种安全、有效的治疗方法。

参考资料

[1] Wong M. Bladder calculi, an evidence-based review[M]. In: Stone disease. The 2nd

International Consultation on Stone Disease. Paris：Editions 21，2008：295-303.

［2］Dhabalia J V，Jain N，Kumar V，et al. Modified technique of percutaneous cystolithotripsy using a new instrument—combined single-step trocar-dilator with self-retaining adjustable access sheath［J］. Urology,2011，77(6)：1304-1307.

［3］Tugcu V，Polat H，Ozbay B，et al. Percutaneous versus transurethral cystolithotripsy［J］. J Endourol. 2009，23(2)：237-241.

［4］Elcioglu O，Ozden H，Guven G，et al. Urinary bladder stone extraction and instruments compared in textbooks of Abul-Qasim Khalaf Ibn Abbas Alzahrawi(Albucasis) (930-1013) and Serefeddin Sabuncuoglu(1385-1470)［J］. J Endourol. 2010，24(9)：1463-1468.

［5］Singh K J and Kaurl J. Comparison of three different endoscopic techniques in management of bladder calculi［J］. Indian J Urol. 2011，27(1)：10-13.

［6］Ener K，Agras K，Aldemir M，et al. The randomized comparison of two different endoscopic techniques in the management of large bladder stones：transurethral use of nephroscope or cystoscope? ［J］. J Endourol. 2009，23(7)：1151-1155.

［7］Kara C，Resorlu B，Cicekbilek I，et al. Transurethral cystolithotripsy with holmium laser under local anesthesia in selected patients［J］. Urology. 2009，74(5)：1000-1003.

［8］Philippou P，Volanis D，Kariotis I，et al. Prospective comparative study of endoscopic management of bladder lithiasis：is prostate surgery a necessary adjunct? ［J］. Urology. 2011，78(1)：43-47.

［9］Shah H N，Hegde S S，Shah J N，et al. Simultaneous transurethral cystolithotripsy with holmium laser enucleation of the prostate：a prospective feasibility study and review of literature［J］. BJU Int. 2007，99(3)：595-600.

［10］Li A，Lu H，Liu S,et al. A Novel Endoscope to Treat Bladder Stone［J］. J Endourol Part B, Videourology. 2011，25；doi：10.1089.

［11］Li A，Ji C，Lu H，et al. Transurethral cystolithotripsy with a novel special endoscope［J］. Urol Res. 2012，40(6)：769-773.

［12］夏术阶. 膀胱结石碎石术［M］//夏术阶. 微创泌尿外科学. 济南：山东科学技术出版社，2007：143-144.

刘思宽　陈蓓珺

附图:

国际泌尿外科学会第 31 届大会

the 31st Congress of the Société Internationale d'Urologi

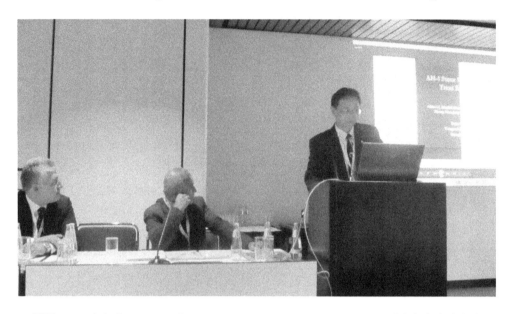

附图 5-1　论文 *AH-1 Stone Removal System to Treat Bladder Stones* 进行视频发言交流

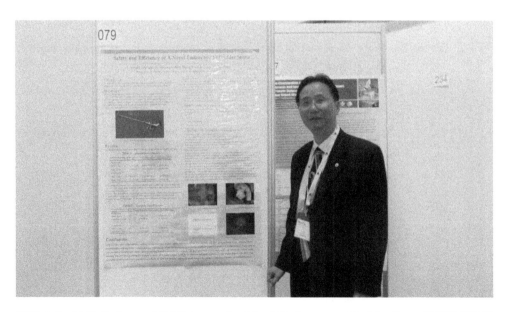

附图 5-2　论文 *Safety and Efficiency of a Novel Endoscope to Bladder Stone* 进行墙报展出

AH-1 型取石系统经尿道治疗大体积膀胱结石的疗效

[摘要] **目的**：目前无论在发展中国家还是在发达国家，用现有器械治疗大体积、大负荷膀胱结石所面临的问题依然没有得到有效解决。AH-1 型取石系统(SRS)主要用于粉碎和摄取结石。本文评估的是 SRS 系统经尿道膀胱碎石治疗不同体积膀胱结石的安全性和有效性。**方法**：由李爱华在 2007 年发明的 SRS 系统由窥镜光源成像系统、手柄、取石钳、碎石通道、液体连续冲洗系统、镜桥、镜鞘等部件组成。2008 年以来，采用 SRS 系统经尿道碎石治疗膀胱结石 163 例。比较不同直径膀胱结石的手术效果，评估手术的疗效和安全性。**结果**：对不同膀胱结石患者的临床资料和取石时间进行了评估。163 例患者中单发性结石为 90 例，在单个结石患者中，A 组结石直径(1.21 ± 0.39) cm，手术时间(9.27 ± 6.95) min；B 组结石直径(2.33 ± 0.30) cm，手术时间(15.25 ± 15.51) min；C 组结石直径(3.27 ± 0.29) cm，手术时间(20.57 ± 9.79) min；D 组结石直径(4.81 ± 0.91) cm，手术时间(58.89 ± 43.43) min。四组间的差异有统计学意义。其中对 109 例(66.87%)伴有 BPH 的患者同时施行 TURP 手术。四组间相比，TURP 手术时间，$P > 0.05$。术中无特殊并发症发生。**结论**：采用 SRS 系统经尿道膀胱碎石可缩短手术时间，降低并发症。是一种安全有效的膀胱结石腔内微创手术方法，更符合伦理学的无伤害原则，并可同时采用 TURP 有效治疗伴发的 BPH。

[关键词] 膀胱结石；经尿道碎石；内镜；AH-1 型取石系统

Efficiency of Transurethral Cystolitholapaxy with the AH-1 Stone Removal System to Large Volume Bladder Stones

ABSTRACT **Background**: The treatment of large volume bladder stones by current equipments continues to be a management problem in both developing and developed countries. AH-1 Stone Removal System(SRS) invented by us is primarily used to crush and retrieve bladder stones. This study evaluated the safety and efficiency of transurethral cystolitholapaxy with SRS for the treatment of bladder stones of variable size. **Methods**: SRS, which was invented by Aihua Li in 2007, composed by endoscope, continuous-flow component, a jaw for stone handling and retrieving, lithotripsy tube, handle, inner sheath and outer sheath. 163 patients with bladder stones were performed by transurethral cystolitholapaxy with SRS since 2008. We compare the surgical outcome to bladder stones of variable size, and evaluate the surgical efficiency and safety. **Results**: Characteristics of patients and stone removal time in variable size were evaluated. 90 patients were with single stone in the 163 patients. To the patients with single stone, stone size was (1.21 ± 0.39) cm and the operating time was (9.27 ± 6.95) min in Group A. Stone size was (2.33 ± 0.30) cm and the operating time was (15.25 ± 15.51) min in Group B. Stone size was (3.27 ± 0.29) cm and the operating time was (20.57 ± 9.79) min in Group C. Stone size was (4.81 ± 0.91) cm and the operating time was (58.89 ± 43.43) min in Group D. The difference was statistically significant between the four groups. Among them, 109(66.87%) patients accompanied with benign prostatic hyperplasia(BPH) were treated by transurethral resection of the prostate(TURP) simultaneously. Compared between the four groups, the difference of the TURP time was not statistically significant, $P > 0.05$. No significant complication was found in the surgical procedure. **Conclusions**: Transurethral cystolitholapaxy with SRS appears to be increased rapidity of the procedure with decreased morbidity. It is a safe and efficient surgical management to bladder stones. This endoscopic surgery best fits the ethics principle of no injury; meanwhile, the accompanied BPH could be effectively treated by TURP simultaneously.

Key words Bladder stone；Transurethral Cystolitholapaxy；Endoscopic surgery；AH-1 Stone Removal System

膀胱结石发病率在发达国家约占泌尿结石的 5%，但是在发展中国家发病率则更高。新颖创新的膀胱结石治疗方法不断出现，但是无论在发展中国家还是在发达国家，用现有器械治疗大体积、大负荷膀胱结石所面临的问题依然没有得到有效解决[1-10]。

治疗膀胱结石最常用的方法是经尿道膀胱结石碎石术。但是用现有的膀胱碎石镜、肾镜、膀胱镜、电切镜或输尿管镜经尿道治疗膀胱结石依然有手术时间长和易损伤膀胱黏膜等问题，存在严重缺陷[4, 11-14]。SRS 系统主要用于粉碎和摄取膀胱结石，是一种具有固定结石、提供碎石通道、自动收集碎石、冲吸碎石、摄取碎石和连续冲洗等功能的多功能内镜[11-13]。早期与采用现有器械的对照组进行比较研究，提示 SRS 系统治疗膀胱结石是安全有效的。本文回顾性探讨过去 7 年采用 RSR 系统治疗的 163 例膀胱结石患者，比较不同体积膀胱结石的手术效果，进一步评估这种手术方法的疗效和安全性。

一、材料与方法

1. 临床资料

2008 年 10 月至 2016 年 4 月共采用 SRS 系统治疗治疗膀胱结石 163 例，其中 98 例伴有 BPH 同时行 TURP。平均年龄 73.5 岁（43～97 岁）。男性 144 例，女性 19 例。根据结石直径大小，163 例患者分为四组。A 组 78 例（结石直径＜2 cm），B 组 54 例（结石直径 2～2.9 cm），C 组 19 例（结石直径 3～3.9 cm），D 组 12 例（结石直径≥4 cm，最大结石直径 6.6 cm）。

2. 手术实施过程和方法

各组均在脊柱麻醉下取截石位，采用国产大族钬激光碎石机，所用功率为

2.6～3.5 J 和 2.0～2.5 Hz。术中,先将内芯置入镜鞘内,然后经尿道将镜鞘插入膀胱,或镜鞘插入尿道后置入镜桥,直视下将镜鞘插入膀胱。入镜后将镜体置入镜鞘内,也可通过镜鞘连接转换器与已经置入膀胱的电切镜外鞘连接。常规膀胱检查、寻找结石。寻及结石后,用取石钳的咬合和下压力固定结石。然后将气压弹道碎石杆或激光碎石光纤通过碎石通道进行碎石。结石粉碎后利用回旋流自动收集碎石,同时应用取石钳夹在镜鞘内拉网状抓取碎石。有大量细小碎石时,镜鞘连接冲吸器,冲吸碎石。结石取净后再行 TURP。单纯结石患者术后 48 h 出院,同时行 TURP 患者术后 5～7 天出院。

对照组[3]经尿道置入 F26 连续冲洗型 Storze 电切镜,寻及结石后用镜鞘固定。镜鞘内置入 F8 Storze 输尿管镜,钬激光碎石后再行 TURP。

3. 统计学方法

对数据资料均以均数±标准误表示,采用两独立样本的 t 检验进行差异显著性检验。假设检验的显著性水平取 $\alpha = 0.05$。

二、结果

1. 患者的基本临床资料

共有 19 例(11.66%)女性患者,A 组 4 例(5.13%),B 组 5 例(9.26%),C 组 3 例(15.79%),D 组 6 例(50.00%)。A 组、B 组与 D 组相比,$P < 0.01$。患者的临床基本资料见表 6-1。

表 6-1 患者临床资料

组别(结石直径范围)	病例 N	结石直径/cm	结石数目	BPH	前列腺体积/ml
A 组(<2 cm)	78	1.31±0.37	9.53±26.4	57	59.1±32.5
B 组(2～2.9 cm)	54	2.31±0.29	2.46±5.56	33	61.4±41.90
C 组(3～3.9 cm)	19	3.23±0.26	1.68±1.34	15	54.9±27.7
D 组(≥4 cm)	12	4.87±0.84	2.42±3.26	4	39.7±18.9
总计	163			109	

多发性结石的直径采用的统计数据为最大结石的直径。四组间相比,前列腺体积的差异无统计学意义,$P>0.05$。

2. 不同体积结石的手术疗效

手术过程中,A组<0.7 cm结石无需碎石,可以直接通过镜鞘顺利取出。0.7~0.9 cm结石也可以通过尿道镜鞘外直接取出。其他体积的结石只能采用先碎石,后用取石钳取出碎石。取石钳夹在抓取碎石时,一次操作可抓取多枚碎石。不同体积结石的手术时间见表6-2。

表6-2　不同体积结石的手术时间

组别(结石直径范围)	取石时间/min	TURP时间/min
A组(<2 cm)	11.92±11.47	34.49±13.54
B组(2~2.9 cm)	17.67±14.60	32.85±10.93
C组(3~3.9 cm)	21.47±10.95	31.8±9.59
D组(≥4 cm)	81.00±59.52	25.0±12.25

取石时间,与A组相比,B组$P<0.05$;C组和D组$P<0.001$,差异有显著意义。与A2组相比,B组和C组$P<0.01$;D组$P<0.001$。与B组相比,C组$P>0.05$;D组$P<0.001$。与C组相比,D组$P<0.01$。TURP手术时间四组间差异无显著意义,$P>0.05$。

3. 单发性结石的手术疗效

163例患者中单发性结石90例,其手术疗效见表6-3。

表6-3　单发结石的取石时间

组别(结石直径范围)	病例 N	结石直径/cm	取石时间/min
A组(<2 cm)	29	1.21±0.39	9.27±6.95
B组(2~2.9 cm)	35	2.33±0.30	15.25±15.51
C组(3~3.9 cm)	14	3.27±0.29	20.57±9.79
D组(≥4 cm)	12	4.81±0.91	58.89±43.43

取石时间与 A 组相比,B 组 $P<0.01$;C 组和 D 组 $P<0.001$,差异有显著意义。与 B 组相比,C 组 $P<0.01$;D 组 $P<0.001$。与 C 组相比,D 组 $P<0.001$。

4. 手术并发症

12 例(7.36%)伴有 BPH 患者,由于增大的中叶致使碎石困难,所以先施行 TURP 或切除中叶,然后再碎石。此时,由于前列腺窝创面渗血,手术视野较模糊。5 例(3.07%)单纯尿道狭窄,尿道扩张后成功插入 SRS 系统碎石成功。2 例(1.23%)<2 cm 结石伴严重尿道狭窄,只能改用输尿管镜进行碎石,此时取石困难,手术时间延长。在 SRS 系统结构改进、可直视下入镜后,上述尿道狭小导致的镜鞘插入困难得到有效地改善。

此外有 4 例(2.46%)低比重结石,结石粉碎后漂浮在膀胱腔内,增加了用取石钳固定结石和摄取结石的困难。3 例高龄 >4 cm 结石,1 例高龄 176 枚 0.7～1.5 cm 结石患者,为手术安全,分两次碎石或 TURP 术。其中 1 例为 92 岁患有 6.6 cm 巨大结石(图 6-1)。膀胱容积小,入镜后膀胱空间小,取石钳无法插入,用力插入后异物钳损坏。

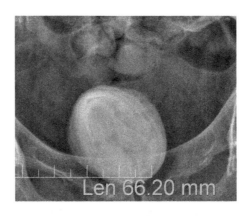

图 6-1 93 岁女性患者患膀胱 6.6 cm 巨大结石,采用 AH-1 型
取石系统成功实施经尿道膀胱结石碎石术

1 例 TURP 术后 10 个月形成的 2.4 cm 结石,其核心由前列腺坏死组织构成。对结石外周粉碎后再用取石钳固定核心坏死组织,钬激光将其切割成 3 块,经尿道取出。

术中无其他特殊并发症发生,无中转开放手术。随访 35.18±20.05 月

（3～72月），期间无手术引起的尿道狭窄及其他相关并发症发生。所有伴有BPH和尿道狭窄的患者均有正常的排尿功能。

三、讨论

现有腔内微创技术仅适用于直径小于 2 cm 的膀胱结石[12]，其主要原因是术中常遇的四大难题：①膀胱空腔大，膀胱结石多大而坚硬，碎石时容易在腔内滑动；②碎石时结石在膀胱腔内跳动，撞击膀胱壁易引起黏膜损伤出血；③结石滑动后钬激光易损伤膀胱黏膜；④结石粉碎后形成大量碎石，加之尿道弯曲，现有设备不易取出；⑤膀胱壁充盈后变薄，容易损伤穿孔；⑥部分内镜无法连续冲洗，视野不清。

应用输尿管镜联合电切镜进行膀胱碎石是一种有效的方法[3]，但是镜鞘固定结石的稳定性远不如 SRS 系统的取石钳，结石过大时常无法固定结石。碎石时，结石经常在膀胱腔内不断滑动，钬激光碎石效率无法有效发挥。用输尿管镜直接碎石，由于输尿管镜进水流量小，又不能持续冲洗，手术视野常模糊不清，容易损伤膀胱黏膜。一旦黏膜损伤出血，视野将更加模糊。加之，膀胱壁充盈后变薄，容易损伤穿孔。因此在处理较大结石时容易损伤膀胱黏膜导致膀胱壁破裂。术中细小结石可采用 Ellick 冲吸器冲吸，也可用电切襻在操作腔内或镜鞘外取出较大碎石。但是取石效率低，容易损坏电切襻。反复使用后容易损坏电切镜上用于锁定电切襻的固定器。本文 2 例由于碎石后产生过多碎石，无法彻底取净，最终改行开放手术。其次，经尿道反复插入电切镜取石会严重损伤尿道黏膜，可导致术后继发性尿道狭窄发生。因此该方法更适用于直径小于 2 cm 的结石。

SRS 系统是一种金属硬性内镜。取石钳位于物镜的前端，由上向下张合，钳夹闭合时，纵观呈圆形，其中央部依然为圆形腔道。取石钳夹片呈框架状，在碎石时易于抓取、固定结石。钳夹的顶端边缘设有阻挡襻后，可在镜鞘内进行拖网式取石，一次可取出多枚结石。金属钳夹可有力地控制 6.4 cm 以下的结石进行碎石操作。镜鞘也可与冲吸器相连冲吸结石。应用流体力学回旋流原理，带有出水孔的镜鞘使 SRS 系统具有自动收集结石的功能。碎石通道位于物镜和光源的下缘，便于在直视下抓取结石进行碎石操作。

术中 SRS 系统可在直视下入镜,结石固定后再进行碎石操作,此时结石无法再在膀胱腔内滑动,用钬激光或气压弹道碎石时碎石效率大幅提高,结石容易粉碎。其次,SRS 系统具有连续冲洗功能,进、出水流量大,故术中可保持清晰视野,便于操作,不易损伤膀胱黏膜。结石粉碎后用 SRS 系统的取石钳在镜鞘内拖网式取石,一次可取出多枚碎石。有较多细小碎石时也可采用冲吸器冲吸取石。同时 SRS 系统的镜鞘内径远大于 F26 连续冲洗型 Storze 电切镜的操作内径,可取出更大碎石。可明显提高取石效率,缩短手术时间。不同于电切镜的电切襻取石方法,SRS 系统的取石钳取石操作一般都是在镜鞘内进行,这样可有效减少镜鞘反复插入尿道导致的尿道黏膜损伤。

膀胱结石多发于男性老年患者,BPH 是男性膀胱结石的主要诱发原因。女性膀胱结石一般多为高龄、长期卧床患者,结石体积通常比较大。SRS 可有效地用于治疗 3 cm 以上的大体积膀胱结石,但是随着结石体积的增大、结石数目的增多,手术难度和时间将会相应延长。但是未发现前列腺体积随着结石体积的增加而增加的现象,因此对于大体积结石的 TURP 手术难度并没有加大,TURP 时间没有延长。对于高龄、高危、结石体积过大和数目过多的患者,可采用分期碎石治疗。对于结石体积过大,膀胱容量过小,取石钳无法顺利插入的患者,不宜强行插入,否则容易损坏取石钳。发生这种情况时,可用输尿管镜、电切镜等其他内镜作为碎石平台,待结石部分粉碎后再使用取石钳。

为避免意外损伤,SRS 系统镜鞘置入膀胱后应直视下插入取石钳。较大结石可在镜鞘外直接取出,但这样的操作对尿道黏膜损伤大,不宜反复使用。术中持续低压冲洗,可保持视野清晰、避免损伤膀胱黏膜。推荐碎石后再行 TURP,这样更易操作。总之,SRS 系统是一种集固定结石、提供碎石通道、自动收集碎石、摄取碎石、冲吸碎石和连续冲洗等功能为一体的多功能内镜。尤其是术中可固定结石、自动收集碎石、一次可摄取多枚碎石。这样可缩短手术时间,提高碎石效率,拓展内镜治疗膀胱结石的手术适应范围。其联合 TURP 用于治疗膀胱结石伴 BPH,是一种安全、有效的治疗方法,但临床病例有待进一步积累。

四、结论

2008 年 1 月至 2016 年 4 月,应用 AH-1 型取石系统经尿道成功治疗 163

例膀胱结石患者。采用SRS系统施行经尿道膀胱碎石取石术是治疗大体积、大负荷膀胱结石的一种安全有效的腔内微创手术。这种手术方法可缩短膀胱结石的手术时间,减少手术并发症。尤其是SRS系统具有固定结石功能,可在碎石时防止结石滑动,提高碎石效率,防止结石滑动造成的损伤出血,碎石后又能快速取净碎石。取石钳在镜鞘内摄取碎石,避免了镜鞘在尿道内的反复进出和碎石对尿道黏膜的摩擦,减少手术操作对尿道的损伤。SRS系统是泌尿外科医生可以选用的膀胱结石手术设备。我们将进一步研发直径更小的,适用于儿童和尿道狭窄的SRS系列产品。

参考资料

［1］ Wong M. Bladder calculi, an evidence-based review［M］. In: Stone disease. The 2nd International Consultation on Stone Disease. Paris: Editions 21, 2008: 295-303.

［2］ Dhabalia J V, Jain N, Kumar V, et al. Modified technique of percutaneous cystolitho-tripsy using a new instrument—combined single-step trocar-dilator with self-retaining adjustable access sheath［J］. Urology. 2011, 77(6):1304-1307.

［3］ Tugcu V, Polat H, Ozbay B, et al. Percutaneous versus transurethral cystolithotripsy ［J］. J Endourol. 2009, 23(2):237-241.

［4］ Elcioglu O, Ozden H, Guven G, et al. Urinary bladder stone extraction and instru-ments compared in textbooks of Abul-Qasim Khalaf Ibn Abbas Alzahrawi(Albucasis) (930-1013) and Serefeddin Sabuncuoglu(1385-1470) ［J］. J Endourol. 2010, 24(9): 1463-1468.

［5］ Singh K J and Kaurl J. Comparison of three different endoscopic techniques in manage-ment of bladder calculi［J］. Indian J Urol. 2011, 27(1): 10-13.

［6］ Ener K, Agras K, Aldemir M, et al. The randomized comparison of two different endo-scopic techniques in the management of large bladder stones: transurethral use of ne-phroscope or cystoscope? ［J］. J Endourol. 2009, 23(7):1151-1155.

［7］ Kara C, Resorlu B, Cicekbilek I, et al. Transurethral cystolithotripsy with holmium la-ser under local anesthesia in selected patients［J］. Urology. 2009, 74(5):1000-1003.

［8］ Philippou P, Volanis D, Kariotis I, et al. Prospective comparative study of endoscopic management of bladder lithiasis: is prostate surgery a necessary adjunct? ［J］. Urology. 2011, 78(1):43-47.

［9］ Shah H N, Hegde S S, Shah J N, et al. Simultaneous transurethral cystolithotripsy with holmium laser enucleation of the prostate: a prospective feasibility study and review of literature[J]. BJU Int. 2007，99(3):595-600.

[10] Li A，Lu H，Liu S,et al. A Novel Endoscope to Treat Bladder Stone[J]. J Endourol Part B，Videourology. 2011，25;doi: 10.1089.

[11] Li A，Ji C,Lu H，et al. Transurethral cystolithotripsy with a novel special endoscope [J]. Urol Res. 2012，40(6):769-773.

[12] 夏术阶. 膀胱结石碎石术[M]//夏术阶.微创泌尿外科学.济南:山东科学技术出版社，2007:143-144.

王　晖　张炳辉

附图

第34届世界腔道泌尿外科大会
The 34th World Congress of Endourology

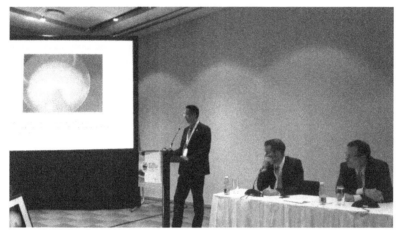

附图6-1 论文 *Efficiency of Transurethral Cystolitholapaxy with AH −1 Stone Removal System to Large Volume Bladder Stones* 进行发言交流

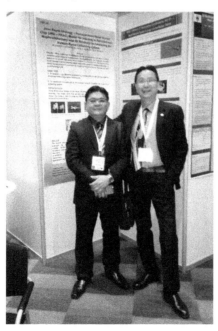

附图6-2 论文 *Efficiency of Transurethral Cystolitholapaxy with AH −1 Stone Removal System to Large Volume Bladder Stones* 进行墙报展出交流

51

第七节

AH-1型取石系统治疗大负荷
膀胱结石病例报告二例

[摘要] **目的:**经尿道膀胱碎石取石术是目前治疗膀胱结石的最好、最常用的方法。然而,目前的医疗设备和手术技术难以满意地用于治疗大负荷膀胱结石。李爱华医生研发了AH-1型取石系统(SRS),其主要功能是用于经尿道粉碎和抓取膀胱结石。本文报告两例大负荷膀胱结石的治疗效果。**病例报告:**报道两例大容量膀胱结石:一例为82岁男性,患有重度良性前列腺增生伴172枚直径0.5~1.5 cm的膀胱结石、多发性膀胱憩室,9枚憩室内结石。另一例为85岁女性,患有一枚直径6.4 cm的巨大膀胱结石。两名患者同时患有严重的全身性疾病,不能实施或拒绝接受膀胱切开取石手术途径和风险。采用SRS系统实施经尿道膀胱碎石取石术,两名患者的膀胱结石被成功碎石后经尿道取出。**结论:**采用SRS系统实施经尿道膀胱碎石取石术可以用于治疗大负荷的膀胱结石。尤其对于高龄、体质过度虚弱、腹部手术疤痕过多,不能实施、接受开放手术或耐受开放手术风险的患者。对于这些患者,采用SRS系统实施经尿道膀胱碎石取石术可能是一种较好的治疗选择。

[关键词] 大负荷膀胱结石;经尿道膀胱结石碎石取石术;AH-1型取石系统

ABSTRACT　Background: Transurethral cystolitholapaxy is probably the better and most common way to manage cystolithiasis. However, the treatment of large volume bladder stones by current medical devices and surgical techniques could be a management problem. AH-1 Stone Removal System

(SRS) invented by us is primarily used to crush and retrieve bladder stones through urethra. The efficiency of two cases of large volume bladder stones were reported in this study. **Case presentation**：We present two cases of large volume bladder stones：one is an 82-year-old man who had serious benign prostatic hyperplasia accompanied with 172 bladder stones in 0. 5～1. 5 cm, multiple bladder diverticulums and 9 diverticular stones. And the other is an 85-year-old woman had a huge bladder stone in 6. 4 cm. The two patients were accompanied with more serious systemic diseases and did not tolerate the surgical risk of cystolithotomy. They were treated by transurethral cystolitholapaxy with SRS and the stones were successfully crushed and retrieved through urethra. **Conclusions**：Transurethral cystolitholapaxy with SRS could be performed to treat large volume bladder stones. Especially for those patients, who are too older or too week and unable to tolerate the surgical risk of open cystolithotomy, transurethral cystitholapaxy with SRS could be considered as a better treatment option.

Key words　Large volume bladder stones；Transurethral cystolitholapaxy；AH-1 Stone Removal System

随着社会老年化,在我国膀胱结石有着稳步增长的趋势。大负荷、大体积的膀胱结石多发生在长期卧床的高龄女性患者和患有严重前列腺增生的老年男性患者。其共有特征性除了有引发膀胱结石的疾病外,表现为年老、体质虚弱、伴有多种全身性疾病。患者和家属有着强烈的微创手术的意愿,希望通过损伤最小、痛苦最轻的方法治愈疾病。同时,由于科学技术的进步,新颖创新的治疗膀胱结石的方法不断出现,但是目前无论在发展中国家还是发达国家,用现有器械治疗大体积、大负荷膀胱结石所面临的问题依然没有取得有效解决[1-8]。现报告两例大负荷、大体积膀胱结石采用 SRS 系统实施经尿道膀胱结石碎石取石术的疗效。一例为重度良性前列腺增生伴 172 枚直径 0.5～1.5 cm 的膀胱结石、多发性膀胱憩室,9 枚憩室内结石。另一例为患有一枚直径6.4 cm 的巨大膀胱结石。两名患者均采用钬激光碎石。

手术器械和方法:手术均在脊柱麻醉下取截石位进行,钬激光碎石所用功率为 2.6～3.5 J 和 2.0～2.5 Hz。具体步骤同第五节和第六节[6-10]。

病 例 报 告 一

一、临床资料

患者：男性，82岁。

主诉：排尿困难伴尿频、尿急一年余。

入院诊断：重度前列腺增生、膀胱多发性结石、膀胱多发性憩室、膀胱憩室内多发性结石、冠心病、慢性心功能不全、慢性阻塞性肺病。

既往病史：冠心病、慢性心功能不全、慢性阻塞性肺病。有支气管哮喘病史10年余，长期进行雾化吸入治疗。

术前检查：

1. KUB平片检查示：前列腺重度增生，突入膀胱。膀胱区增生前列腺周边多发性致密影。

2. 腹部CT和盆腔MRI：前列腺重度增生，突入膀胱。体积大小约为5.31 cm×6.78 cm×4.01 cm，慢性膀胱炎伴多发憩室，膀胱多发结石，憩室内多发性结石。结石直径约0.5～1.5 cm。

3. 腹部彩超：轻度脂肪肝，肝脏多发囊肿。

4. 胸片：两肺纹理增多，主动脉硬化。

美国麻醉学会评分（ASA）：Ⅲ分。

术前影像学资料：

1. 术前KUB显示膀胱多发性结石伴前列腺重度增生（图7-1）。

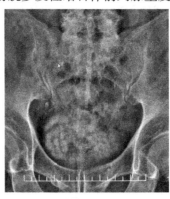

图 7-1

2. 如图 7-2 所示,术前 CT 扫描显示前列腺重度增生、中叶向膀胱腔内严重突出,膀胱腔内有大量结石。膀胱壁多发性憩室,右后壁憩室内多发性结石。膀胱壁内多发性结石。(a)图箭头所示为突入膀胱腔内的增生前列腺;(b)图箭头所示为膀胱憩室内多发结石。

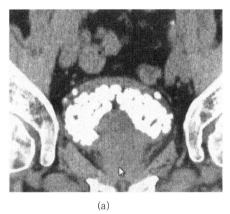
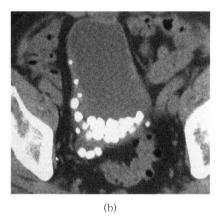

(a)　　　　　　　　　　　　　　　(b)

图 7-2

3. 如图 7-3 所示,术前 MRI 显示膀胱多发性结石伴前列腺重度增生向膀胱腔内严重突出、膀胱后壁憩室内多发性结石。(a)图箭头所示为膀胱后壁憩室内多发结石;(b)图箭头所示为严重突出的前列腺中叶。

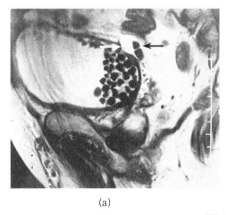
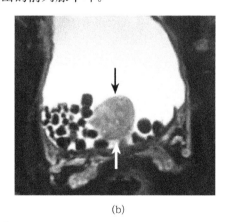

(a)　　　　　　　　　　　　　　　(b)

图 7-3

二、手术方法

患者拒绝耻骨上膀胱切开取石术和经皮耻骨上膀胱穿刺碎石术,故采用

AH-1 型取石系统实施经尿道膀胱结石碎石取石术联合 TURP 术。手术分两步完成。在第一次实施经尿道内镜手术时,对较大结石粉碎后采用 AH-1 型取石系统取出,较小结石可直接取出,共取出 130 枚,然后再实施 TURP 术。总手术时间 90 min,取石时间 60 min,TURP 手术时间 30 min。术后 9 天进行第二次手术。采用上述方法取出膀胱残余结石 33 枚,在 3 个膀胱憩室内取出结石 9 枚。总手术时间 60 min。术中,<0.7 cm 结石无需碎石,可用 AH-1 型取石系统的取石钳通过镜鞘内直接取出;0.7~1.0 cm 结石可用取石钳通过尿道取出;>1 cm 结石应先碎石,粉碎后再取出。两次手术共取出结石 172 枚(图 7-4)。手术过程中未发现有特殊意义的并发症。

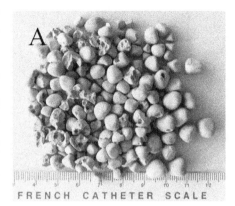

图 7-4　在膀胱内和膀胱壁憩室内取出的 172 枚结石

三、术后 CT 复查

术后 CT 扫描显示膀胱腔内结石已经完全清除,但是膀胱壁内还留有少量残余结石(图 7-5)。

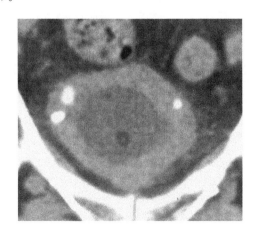

图 7-5　术后 CT 复查,显示箭头所示处为膀胱壁内残余结石

病例报告二

一、临床资料

患者：女性，85 岁。

主诉：尿频、尿急、尿痛伴间歇性肉眼血尿 4 年余。

入院诊断：膀胱巨大结石伴严重尿路感染、宫颈癌术后、2 型糖尿病、右肾积水、低血钾、胆囊结石。

既往病史：20 年前患有宫颈癌，为治疗宫颈癌已实施腹部手术 3 次。术后曾进行多次放疗和化疗。15 年前因放疗导致二下肢动脉闭塞坏疽行双侧下肢截肢术（图 7-6）。术后患者长期卧床。有糖尿病史 15 年，目前进行药物治疗，血糖控制尚佳。

术前检查：

1. KUB 检查示：膀胱区巨大高密度影，直径约 6.4 cm，膀胱结石考虑。

2. 胸片：两肺纹理增多，主动脉硬化。

ASA 评分：Ⅲ分。

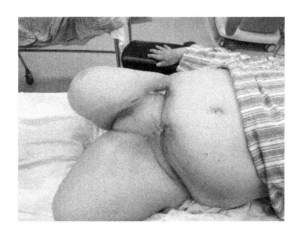

图 7-6　腹部的三次手术和多次放疗导致患者的腹壁布满了手术疤痕和放射性皮肤损伤疤痕，且二下肢已施行高位截肢

术前影像学资料：术前KUB显示膀胱内巨大结石（图7-7）。

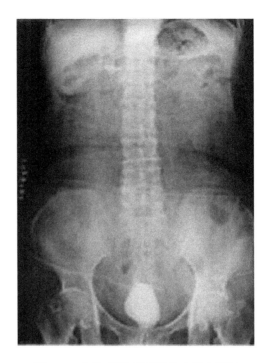

图7-7　术前KUB显示膀胱内巨大结石

二、手术方法

患者腹部因宫颈癌已经实施过三次手术和多次放疗，导致患者的腹壁布满了手术疤痕和放射性皮肤损伤疤痕，故采用AH-1型取石系统实施经尿道膀胱结石碎石取石术。手术一次完成，手术时间98 min。手术过程中未发现有特殊意义的并发症。

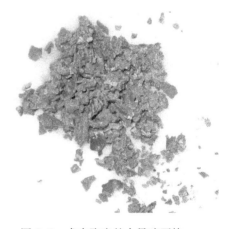

图7-8　术中取出的大量碎石块

三、术后KUB复查

术后KUB显示膀胱无结石残留(图7-9)。

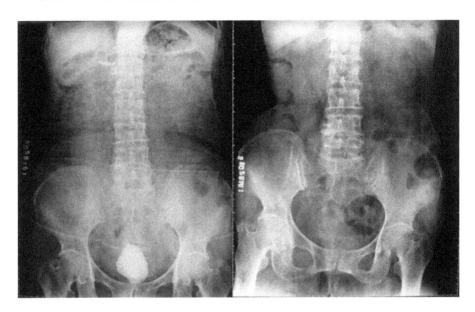

图 7-9　术后KUB显示膀胱无结石残留

讨论

膀胱结石在发展中国家是一种常见的的疾病,在临床上通常会出现下尿路梗阻、尿路感染的不同临床表现,引起患者的不适。在我国多见于高龄前列腺增生患者和长期卧床的老年女性。在过去的几十年中,随着科学技术的进步,各种新颖的膀胱结石治疗方法不断涌现。虽然最常用和最好的膀胱结石治疗方法依然是经尿道膀胱碎石术,由于利用尿道这一人体自然通道进入膀胱进行碎石,因此对人体损伤较小,尤其是老年患者。

但是利用膀胱镜、输尿管镜、肾镜或电切镜等现有内镜设备作为经尿道碎石平台实施经尿道膀胱结石碎石术,由于手术时无法克服的关键性和共性的技术难题,手术时间长、并发症多。这些尚未解决的问题有:①膀胱空腔大结石容易在腔内滑动,因此膀胱结石不易粉碎,碎石效率不高;②碎石时结石在膀胱腔内跳动,撞击膀胱壁易引起黏膜损伤出血;③结石滑动后或破裂时钬激光易损伤膀胱黏膜;④在治疗多发性膀胱结石,或大体积膀胱结石粉碎后形成大量碎石时,现有异物钳或电切襻等设备不易快速取出碎石,尤其是男性患者,由于尿道弯曲而细长更不易取出;⑤膀胱壁充盈后变薄,容易损伤穿孔。因此无论在发展中国家还是在发达国家,用现有器械治疗大体积、大负荷膀胱结石所面临的问题依然没有取得有效解决[1-8]。

李爱华医生研发的 SRS 系统是一种集固定结石、提供碎石通道、自动收集碎石、摄取碎石、冲吸碎石和连续冲洗等功能为一体的多功能内镜。尤其是术中可固定结石、自动收集碎石、一次可摄取多枚碎石。与现有方法比较,可缩短手术时间,提高碎石效率,减少意外损伤,拓展内镜治疗膀胱结石的手术适应范围[6-8]。

病例一是一名 82 岁患有重度前列腺增生,伴有 172 枚 0.5~1.5 cm 的膀胱结石、多发性膀胱憩室、多发性膀胱憩室内结石的患者。根据目前的医疗设备和膀胱结石的治疗技术,只有通过开放手术才能取出这么多的膀胱结石和憩室内结石。然而,患者拒绝开放手术,同时其患有严重的冠心病、慢性肺部梗阻性疾病和哮喘,耐受手术风险的能力也很差。考虑到既要粉碎和取出 172 枚膀胱结石,同时还要切除增大的前列腺,将会耗去大量手术时间,因此根据患者的病情制定了分两步实施手术操作的治疗方案。第一次手术经尿道采用 AH-1型取石系统尽量粉碎和取出较多的膀胱结石,再实施 TURP 手术切除增生前列腺;第二次手术时已无增大前列腺的阻挡,因此能经尿道顺利粉碎和取出大量的膀胱残余结石,然后经仔细检查,又取出 3 个膀胱憩室内的 9 枚结石[7-10]。手术方案成功实施,患者对手术过程和疗效十分满意。

病例二是一名 85 岁患有 6.4 cm 膀胱巨大结石的老年女性。腹部有以往三次手术留下的手术创伤和疤痕,以及多次放疗对组织造成的放射性损伤和疤痕。加之,患者有 15 年的糖尿病史。采用耻骨上膀胱切开取石术或经皮耻骨上膀胱穿刺碎石术治疗,可能会因手术疤痕和组织黏连使手术操作变得十分困难,术后也可能因组织放射性损伤导致切口长期不愈。同时,患者由于医源性的疾病已经行双侧下肢截肢术。故选用 AH-1 型取石系统经尿道碎石术,一次粉碎,取净 6.4 cm的膀胱结石。手术过程没有给患者带来更多的痛苦,没有在腹部留下更多的疤痕。这种内镜治疗膀胱结石的方法更符合医学伦理学的无伤害原则[6-8]。

结论

两例病例报告显示,采用 AH-1 型取石系统和钬激光经尿道膀胱碎石术治疗大负荷、大体积膀胱结石可取得满意疗效。在治疗多发性、大体积的膀胱结石时,可选用 AH-1 型取石系统和钬激光行经尿道膀胱碎石术进行治疗。特别是对那些不愿接受有创手术或者承受开放手术的患者,采用 AH-1 型取石系统经尿道膀胱碎石取石术可以被视为一种更好的治疗选择。

参考资料

[1] Zhao J, Shi L, Gao Z, Liu Q, Wang K, Zhang P. Minimally invasive surgery for patients with bulky bladder stones and large benign prostatic hyperplasia simultaneously: a novel design. Urol Int. 2013,91:31-37.

[2] Tan YK, Gupta DM, Weinberg A, Matteis A J, Kotwal S, Gupta M. Minimally invasive percutaneous management of large bladder stones with a laparoscopic entrapment bag. J Endourol. 2014,28:61-64.

[3] Torricelli F C, Mazzucchi E, Danilovic A, Coelho R F, Srougi M. Surgical management of bladder stones: literature review. Rev Col Bras Cir. 2013;40:227-233.

[4] De S, Sarkissian C, Marchinni G, Monga M. Concurrent stone stabilization improves ultrasonic and pneumatic efficacy during cystolithopaxy: an in vitro analysis. Int Braz J Urol. 2015, 41:134-138.

[5] Wu J H, Yang K, Liu Q, Yang S Q, Xu Y. Combined usage of Ho: YAG laser with monopolar resectoscope in the treatment of bladder stone and bladder outlet obstruction. Pak J Med Sci. 2014, 30:908-913.

[6] Li A, Lu H, Liu S, Feng Zhang, Xiaoqiang Qian, Hui Wang. A Novel Endoscope to Treat Bladder Stone. J Endourol Part B, Videourology 2011, 25(2):doi: 10.1089.

[7] Li A, Lu H, Ji C, Liu S, Zhang F, Qian X,et al. Transurethral cystolithotripsy with a novel special endoscope. Urol Res. 2012,40:769-773.

[8] Li A, Ji C, Wang H, Lang G, Lu H, Liu S,et al. Transurethral Cystolitholapaxy with the AH-1 Stone Removal System for the Treatment of Bladder Stones of Variable Size. BMC Urology. 2015, 15:9.

[9] Li A, Lu H, Liu S, Zhang F, Qian X, Wang H. Effect of Ageing on the Efficiency of TUVRP. The Aging Male. 2012,15:263-266.

[10] Li A, Zhang Y, Lu H, Zhang F, Liu S, Wang H, et al. Living Status in Patients over 85 Years of Age after TUVRP. The Aging Male. 2013,16:191-194.

王　晖　李爱华

第八节
AH-1 型取石系统与国内外现有同类技术的综合比较

一、与国内外现有膀胱碎石镜和替代内镜比较

目前用于经尿道治疗膀胱结石的内镜有膀胱碎石镜,替代内镜设备有:①膀胱镜;②输尿管镜;③肾镜;④电切镜;⑤上述内镜配套的异物钳。这些替代内镜仅适用于治疗直径小于 2 cm 的膀胱结石,主要原因是术中常遇的五大难题尚未解决:①膀胱大结石多坚硬,膀胱空腔大,结石易滑动,不易被粉碎;②男性尿道长而弯曲,多发性结石或粉碎后形成的大量碎石不易取出;③经尿道反复取石易损伤尿道;④无法连续冲洗,视野不清;⑤膀胱壁充盈后变薄,容易损伤穿孔。因此,国内外各种教科书依然仅将直径小于 2 cm 的膀胱结石纳入经尿道腔镜微创碎石技术治疗的手术适应证范围。

1. 碎石效率

现有膀胱碎石镜采用机械力学原理,通过碎石钳咬合力的机械挤压将结石粉碎。但是由于操作时很难将结石粉碎,粉碎后也很难取净,并且在粉碎结石的过程中容易损伤膀胱、尿道黏膜,故临床上已很少使用。

电切镜、膀胱镜、输尿管镜和肾镜替代用于治疗膀胱结石,可为碎石设备提供操作通道。碎石时,结石在膀胱腔内不断滑动,碎石效率无法有效发挥。目前,国内有较多医疗机构创新采用电切镜经尿道进行膀胱碎石治疗。但是通过电切镜电极插孔插入碎石光纤后进行碎石,结石无法固定,激光光纤活动度过

大,碎石效率低。若用电切镜镜鞘固定结石,在电切镜镜鞘内再用输尿管镜进行碎石,当结石过大时,镜鞘常无法固定结石。

AH-1型取石系统是将结石固定后再采用钬激光或气压弹道设备进行碎石,结石容易粉碎,可大幅提高碎石效率,缩短手术时间。

2. 取石效率

目前,各种膀胱、输尿管异物钳只能摄取体积较小的碎石,结石粉碎后缺乏有效的手段快速清除碎石。用电切镜的冲洗器冲吸碎石,只能盲目地冲吸细小碎石,很难将结石全部取净。虽然采用电切镜的环状电切襻可摄取较大碎石,但是反复直接通过尿道摄取碎石,会严重损伤尿道黏膜,导致术后尿道狭窄的发生。同时,反复使用电切襻摄取碎石对昂贵的电切襻和电切镜操作件上的电极固定卡扣的损耗是显而易见的。碎石过多时,操作难度和手术时间将明显增加。

AH-1型取石系统利用回旋流自动收集碎石后,取石钳在镜鞘内拖网状抓取碎石,一次可取出多枚碎石,提高了取石效率,缩短了手术时间。

3. 手术安全性

用现有替代内镜碎石,术中不能持续冲洗,手术视野常模糊不清,容易损伤膀胱黏膜。一旦黏膜损伤出血,视野将更加模糊。加之,膀胱壁充盈后变薄,容易损伤穿孔。因此处理较大结石时容易损伤膀胱黏膜,导致膀胱壁破裂。用电切镜反复经尿道取石,容易损伤尿道黏膜,导致术后继发性尿道狭窄发生。反复使用容易损坏电切襻和电切镜上用于锁定电切襻的固定器。

AH-1型取石系统可在直视下插入膀胱,避免盲插的意外损伤。其具有连续冲洗功能,进、出水流量大,术中可保持视野清晰,不易误伤膀胱黏膜。取石钳在镜鞘内拖网状摄取碎石,有较多细小碎石时可采用冲吸器冲吸取石,有效避免了反复经尿道取石对尿道的损伤,减少了术后继发性尿道狭窄发生。

4. 市场价格

AH-1型取石系统市场售价低于经尿道膀胱碎石取石的现有替代内镜(如

膀胱碎石镜、电切镜、膀胱镜、输尿管镜、肾镜)的市场售价。

二、与国际最先进碎石系统比较

AH-1 型取石系统与瑞士 EMS 碎石清石系统(EMS)经尿道膀胱碎石的效价比见表 8-1。EMS 是目前国际上最先进的专用碎石取石系统,它包括气压弹道碎石和超声碎石设备以及负压吸引系统,具有碎石和吸取碎石两项功能。AH-1 型取石系统具有固定结石、摄取碎石、冲吸碎石、连续冲洗、提供碎石通道和自动搜集碎石六项功能,并可通过镜鞘转换器与各种类型的电切镜外鞘连接,通用性强,可使用气压弹道或效率更高的钬激光碎石设备。EMS 需要将结石粉碎成粉末状后才能吸出,取石效率与 AH-1 型取石系统存在巨大差距。EMS 无固定结石功能,用于经尿道膀胱碎石时碎石效率低下。

表 8-1　AH-1 型取石系统与瑞士 EMS 碎石清石系统经尿道膀胱碎石的效价比

	AH-1 型取石系统系统	EMS 系统
碎石方式	气压弹道、钬激光	气压弹道、超声
固定结石	能、碎石效率高	不能、碎石效率低
取石方式	取石钳夹一次抓取多枚结石	负压吸取细小碎石
	冲洗器冲吸细小碎石	
取出碎石体积	颗粒粗大	颗粒细小
	鞘内<8.2 mm、鞘外更粗大	<3 mm、同时碎石时更细小
碎石时间	耗时短	耗时长
配套设备	利用现有碎石设备	利用现有内镜

AH-1 型取石系统取出的碎石粗大,对于直径小于 7 mm 的结石或碎石可直接通过镜鞘取出(图 8-1)。EMS 系统取出的碎石呈泥沙样(直径小于 3 mm),对于同样 AH-1 型能取出的直径小于 7 mm 结石或碎石则必须要进行进一步的粉碎,直至直径小于 3 mm,呈泥沙样时方能通过 EMS 的负压系统吸出,因此要消耗更多的能量和时间进行碎石(图 8-2)。

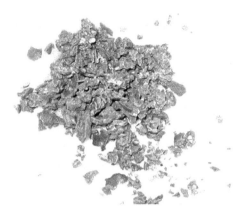
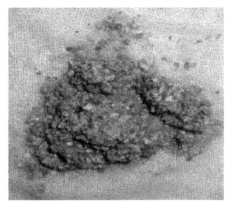

图 8-1　AH-1 型取石系统取出的粗大碎石　　图 8-2　EMS 系统取出的泥沙样碎石

三、入选上海卫生系统先进适宜技术推广项目

AH-1 型取石系统用于经尿道治疗膀胱结石,其性能和价格优于现有设备,综合技术适用于我国的经济现状。该项治疗方法经济实用、操作技术门槛和配套设备要求低。因此适用于在我国二级以上医院推广。尤其在二级医院,可就地解决结石体积较大、年老体弱膀胱结石患者的治疗需求。得到了中华泌尿外科学会主委孙颖浩教授,中国男科医师协会会长夏术阶教授的推荐。2013年入选上海卫生系统先进适宜技术推广项目(编号:2013SY063)。目前在国内已经有数十家医院将 AH-1 型取石系统应用于临床,经尿道治疗膀胱结石。

四、国际泌尿外科学会引用推荐

由国际泌尿外科学会(the Société Internationale d'Urologie)和国际泌尿外科疾病咨询委员会(International Consultation on Urological Diseases)联合编写的 *Stone Disease* 一书已于 2015 年出版。该泌尿外科疾病诊疗咨询指南类专著中引用推荐了 AH-1 型取石系统在膀胱结石治疗中的应用。术中较详细地介绍了AH-1型取石系统的技术结构、临床功能和经尿道膀胱碎石的初期手术疗效,并列表与现有的其他手术方法进行了疗效比较。

2015 年在国际泌尿外科学会第 35 届大会（the 35th Congress of the Société Internationale d'Urologie）期间，应学术报告会主席 Lukman Hakim 教授的邀请，论文 *Transurethral Cystolitholapaxy with the AH-1 Stone Removal System to Treat Large Volume Bladder Stones* 在会议主办的泌尿外科适宜新技术学术报告会（the Symposium on Affordable New Technologies in Urology）上进行了推广演讲，展示交流了这项发展中国家也能购买支付的先进适宜设备和技术。

李爱华　王　晖　刘思宽

附图:

国际泌尿外科学会第 35 届大会
the 35th Congress of the Société Internationale d'Urologie

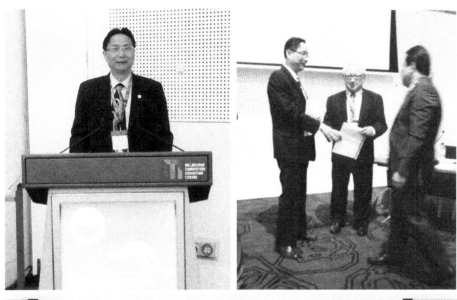

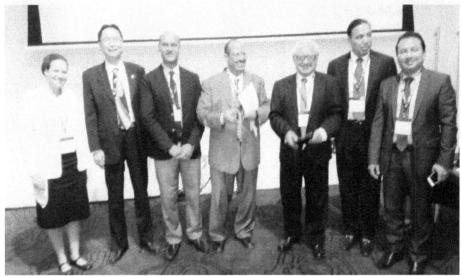

附图 8-1　论文 *Transurethral Cystolitholapaxy with the AH-1 Stone Removal System to Treat Large Volume Bladder Stones* 进行墙报展出,并在会议主办的第 4 届泌尿外科先进适宜新技术推广论坛(the 4th Symposium on Affordable New Technologies in Urology)发言,进行推广交流

第九节
发表论文和学术交流

一、发表论文

1. Transurethral Cystolitholapaxy with the AH-1 Stone Removal System for the Treatment of Bladder Stones of Variable Size. BMC Urology. 2015，15:9.

2. Transurethral cystolithotripsy with a novel special endoscope. Urol Res. 2012,40(6):769-773.

3. A novel endoscope to treat bladder stone. J Endourol Part B，Videourology. 2011，25;doi:10.1089(视频论文).

4. Safety and Efficiency of a novel endoscope to bladder stone. Urology. 2011,76(S3A):S369.

5. AH-1 stone removal system to treat bladder stones. Urology. 2011，76(S3A): S172.

6. Transurethral Cystolitholapaxy with the AH-1 Stone Removal System to Treat Large Volume Bladder stones. World Journal of Urology 2015,33 (S1)35th Congress of the Société Internationale d'Urologie—SIU ABSTRACT BOOK:218-219.

7. AH-1 型取石系统经尿道膀胱碎石的疗效评估. 现代泌尿外科杂志. 2013,18(5):437-440.

二、学术交流

1. 国际泌尿外科学会第 31 届大会(the 31st Congress of the Société Internationale d'Urologie)，论文 *AH-1 Stone Removal System to Treat Bladder Stones* 进行视频发言交流。论文 *Safety and Efficiency of a Novel Endoscope to Bladder Stone* 进行墙报展出，德国柏林，2011 年。

2. 国际泌尿外科学会第 35 届大会(the 35th Congress of the Société Internationale d'Urologie)论文 *Transurethral Cystolitholapaxy with the AH-1 Stone Removal System to Treat Large Volume Bladder Stones* 进行墙报展出，并在会议主办的第 4 届泌尿外科先进适宜新技术论坛(The 4th Symposium on Affordable New Technologies in Urology)发言推广交流，澳大利亚墨尔本，2015 年。

3. 第 34 届世界腔道泌尿外科大会(The 34th World Congress of Endourology)论文 *Efficiency of Transurethral Cystolitholapaxy with AH-1 Stone Removal System to Large Volume Bladder Stones* 发言推广交流，南非开普敦，2016 年。

第十节
科研项目、授权专利和学术奖励

一、科研项目

1. 2006 年、2010 年获杨浦区重点学科建设主攻项目资助。

2. 2012 年获杨浦区人才专项发展基金（鼎元资金）高层人才科研成果转化类资金资助。

3. 2013 年入选上海卫生系统先进适宜技术推广项目，编号：2013SY063。

二、授权专利

1. 膀胱肾盂取石镜。国际发明专利 PCT，编号：WO2009/092182282。

2. 膀胱肾盂取石镜。发明专利 ZL2008132850.4。

3. 用于膀胱肾盂取石镜的钳夹。实用新型专利 ZL200820054918.4。

4. 冲洗结构改良型膀胱肾盂取石镜。实用新型专利 ZL200820155132.1。

5. 镜鞘壁上设有出水孔的膀胱肾盂取石镜。实用新型专利 ZL200920072709.7。

6. 用于膀胱肾盂取石镜的镜桥。实用新型专利 ZL201220007532.4。

7. 用于膀胱肾盂取石镜的多用途镜鞘转换器。实用新型专利 ZL201520141769.5。

三、学术奖励

1. 2010 年获上海医学科技三等奖。
2. 2012 年获第二十四届上海市优秀发明选拔赛职工技术创新成果铜奖。
3. 2013 年入围 2013 年吴阶平泌尿外科医学奖。
4. 2016 年获 2014 年度上海市技术发明奖三等奖。
5. 2015 年度华夏医学科技奖三等奖。

四、国际诊疗指南书籍引用推荐

国际泌尿外科学会(the Société Internationale d'Urologie)和国际泌尿外科疾病咨询委员会(International Consultation on Urological Diseases)联合编写的 *Stone Disease* 引用推荐。

附录1

上海市卫计委有关上海卫生系统
先进适宜技术推广项目的文件

上海市卫生和计划生育委员会文件

沪卫计科教〔2013〕19号

关于下达
上海卫生系统先进适宜技术推广项目的通知

各有关单位：

为提高基层医疗卫生机构卫生技术应用能力和综合服务能力，为城乡居民提供优质、合理、安全的医疗卫生技术，提高人民健康水平，根据《关于加强本市卫生系统学科建设与人才培养工作的指导意见》（沪卫科教〔2012〕6号），启动先进适宜技术推广项目。经专家评审，确定将"急性早幼粒细胞白血病及弥漫大B细胞性淋巴瘤在基层医院的规范化治疗"等75个项目列入先进适宜技术推广项目，项目研究周期均为三年，每个项目资助经费50万元，研究经费立项后拨付50%，中期评估后拨付40%，验收合格后拨付10%，各单位可根据实际情况对项目进行配套资助。

请各项目承担单位督促项目组严格按照医学伦理、生物安全以及知识产权的有关要求开展研究，并根据科研课题管理要求，做好项目的组织实施和管理工作。我委将定期组织项目督导。

附件：上海卫生系统先进适宜技术推广项目立项清单

上海市卫生和计划生育委员会

2013 年 12 月 1 日

上海卫生系统先进适宜技术推广项目立项清单

序号	项目名称	工作单位	负责人
1	急性早幼粒细胞白血病及弥漫大B细胞性淋巴瘤在基层医院的规范化治疗	上海交通大学医学院附属瑞金医院	李军民
2	脑卒中康复社区适宜技术的推广	华东医院	郑洁皎
3	抑郁症的重复经颅磁刺激治疗技术	上海市精神卫生中心	王继军
4	甲状腺乳头状微癌的诊治规范	复旦大学附属肿瘤医院	嵇庆海
5	超声定量肝脏脂肪含量技术的推广应用及脂肪肝相关代谢紊乱的规范化管理	复旦大学附属中山医院	高鑫
6	糖尿病自我管理与支持的技术推广	复旦大学	傅华
7	光动力治疗HPV相关性疾病适宜技术规范推广研究	上海市皮肤病医院	王秀丽
8	SPECT/CT融合图像技术的临床应用	复旦大学附属中山医院	石洪成
9	国际标准化放射治疗质量控制技术	复旦大学附属肿瘤医院	章真
10	微创技术在胃肠道肿瘤早诊早治中的应用	上海交通大学医学院附属瑞金医院	郑民华
11	海洛因依赖者预防复发心理行为干预技术	上海市精神卫生中心	赵敏
12	精神分裂症社区防治预警及综合干预技术	上海市精神卫生中心	蔡军
13	多学科团队在结直肠癌肝转移诊疗中的应用推广	复旦大学附属中山医院	许剑民
14	平衡导引与手法防治青少年特发性脊柱侧凸症的推广应用研究	上海中医药大学附属龙华医院	胡志俊
15	糖尿病慢性并发症筛查适宜技术的推广	上海市第六人民医院	贾伟平
16	肾上腺疾病早期筛查适宜技术推广	上海交通大学医学院附属瑞金	王卫庆

		医院	
17	系统性血管炎标准化筛查与诊断在基层医院的应用	上海交通大学医学院附属瑞金医院	陈楠
18	中医护理技术在肿瘤患者症状群管理中的应用	上海中医药大学附属龙华医院	周文琴
19	微血管减压治疗三叉神经痛和面肌痉挛的技术进展与推广	上海交通大学医学院附属新华医院	李世亭
20	剖宫产术后子宫切口愈合不良（切口憩室）微创手术治疗的研究	复旦大学附属妇产科医院	华克勤
21	肌电图的术中检测在周围神经损伤中的应用技术	复旦大学附属华山医院	田东
22	中枢性偏瘫上肢功能恢复的外科新技术开发与推广	复旦大学附属华山医院	徐文东
23	胸腔镜（VATS)肺叶/肺段切除术治疗 I 期非小细胞肺癌	上海市肺科医院	姜格宁
24	恶性脑肿瘤筛查、早期诊断系统的研究与推广	上海交通大学医学院附属仁济医院	邱永明
25	电子视频多功能喉镜(HPHJ-A 型）在气管插管中的应用	上海长征医院	石学银
26	划痕术治疗酒渣鼻	上海中医药大学附属曙光医院	何翔
27	基于个体综合评价体系的早期肾癌射频消融术	上海交通大学医学院附属仁济医院	黄翼然
28	腹腔镜技术儿童斜疝手术中的应用和推广	上海交通大学医学院附属新华医院	吴晔明
29	社区推广糖尿病教育 DVD 和有氧运动计步器的计划	复旦大学附属华山医院	胡仁明
30	住院患者高危风险预警预控技术	上海市第十人民医院	施雁、戴琳峰
31	超声引导神经阻滞在老年患者麻醉中的应用	上海市第六人民医院	王爱忠

32	国产神经阻滞针机器引导的术后镇痛技术推广应用	上海市同济医院	余斌
33	胸腔镜技术在胸部疾病诊治中的推广应用	上海市胸科医院	茅腾
34	环孢素 A 对反复自然流产的保胎作用及其安全性评价	复旦大学附属妇产科医院	杜美蓉
35	肝脏移植预后相关遗传标志体系建立及其临床应用	上海市第一人民医院	彭志海
36	用于非小细胞型肺癌早期诊断的 99mTc 标记 SSTA 放射受体显像试标准化技术的推广应用	上海市第十人民医院	吕中伟
37	严重创伤院内一体化救治系列技术研究与推广	第二军人学附属长征医院	林兆奋
38	儿童国际创伤生命支持急救技术规范	上海交通大学医学院附属新华医院	潘曙明
39	群发、危重伤全程一体化救治技术规范化应用	上海市东方医院	李钦传
40	手法复位诊治 Bppv 的推广应用	上海市第六人民医院	殷善开
41	全眼球中期保存技术和角膜移植联合白内障手术相关技术推广及应用	上海市第十人民医院	盛敏杰
42	情绪障碍中学生行为激活团体干预学校应用推广效果评估	上海市精神卫生中心	程文红
43	肘关节损伤与功能障碍的规范化治疗平台建设	上海市第六人民医院	范存义
44	石氏针药结合治疗急性踝关节扭伤的推广应用研究	上海中医药大学附属曙光医院	赵咏芳
45	大肠癌致急性肠梗阻的内镜金属支架引流技术	复旦大学附属中山医院	钟芸诗
46	光动力治疗 CIN 逆转宫颈癌前病变	上海市第十人民医院	许青
47	结节病与菌阴结核病鉴别诊断新技术的推广应用	上海市肺科医院	李惠萍
48	慢性肾脏病早期干预技术与规范的推广应用	复旦大学附属中山医院	滕杰
49	13C-尿素呼气试验检测幽门螺杆菌操作规程的推广	华东医院	保志军
50	拖线疗法治疗复杂性肛瘘基层推广应用研究	上海中医药大学附属龙华医院	曹永清

51	家庭医生移动信息平台	上海市徐汇区斜土街道社区卫生服务中心	吴克明
52	智能听力筛查系统在学龄前儿童听力筛查中的推广应用	上海交通大学医学院附属新华医院	吴皓
53	胰腺囊性肿瘤数据库的建立及其在二级预防中的应用	复旦大学附属中山医院	吴文川
54	基于内镜的胃癌早期诊断与微创规范化治疗	复旦大学附属中山医院	姚礼庆
55	系列改良盆底功能重建手术的应用推广	上海市同济医院	童晓文
56	新生儿复杂先心病围生期诊断和治疗关键技术的建立和应用	上海交通大学医学院附属上海儿童医学中心	张海波
57	一次性颅骨整形性外减压术	上海市浦东新区浦南医院	刘卫东
58	24 小时眼压监测对青光眼诊断、治疗的评价作用	复旦大学附属眼耳鼻喉科医院	孙兴怀
59	感染标志物的手工高通量 ELISA 筛查平台的建立与应用	上海市儿童医院	张泓
60	腔内联合植入碘-125 粒子条及支架治疗门脉、下腔静脉及胆道恶性梗阻	复旦大学附属中山医院	罗剑钧
61	急性有机磷农药中毒标准化治疗方案的推广应用	上海市第一人民医院	王瑞兰
62	通过 EDC 系统对川崎病合并冠状动脉病变随访的应用与评价	上海市儿童医院	黄敏
63	一种新型内镜经尿道膀胱碎石的临床推广应用	上海市杨浦区中心医院	李爱华
64	多通道呼吸道病毒检测在社区获得性呼吸道感染临床诊断中的应用	上海市公共卫生临床中心	周晓明
65	上海地区糖化血红蛋白检测结果一致性和互认研究	复旦大学附属中山医院	潘柏申
66	进一步提高超声造影诊断水平并促进其规范化应用	上海市第十人民医院	徐辉雄
67	应用磁共振三维成像测量多囊肾病患者肾脏及囊肿体积	第二军医大学附属长征医院	梅长林

68	TRST 及亲神经性 NMDAR 抗体在神经梅毒早期诊断中的应用	上海市皮肤病医院	周平玉
69	ERP 系列诊疗新技术在精神分裂症中的推广应用研究	上海市精神卫生中心	陈兴时
70	大黄对创伤后全身炎症反应和胃肠功能衰竭的治疗作用	第二军医大学附属长征医院	陈德昌
71	腹腔镜下子宫动脉阻断技术治疗子宫肌瘤	上海市杨浦区中心医院	程忠平
72	针药结合治疗脂肪性肝病的临床运用	上海市长宁区中心医院	张琴
73	儿童常见血液病的早期诊断与规范化诊疗技术推广	上海市同济医院	谢晓恬
74	上海市住院医师规范化培训政策评估及推广研究	复旦大学	黄葭燕
75	磁共振功能影像技术在卵巢癌诊断和鉴别诊断中的应用	复旦大学附属金山医院	强金伟

Li et al. BMC Urology (2015) 15:9
DOI 10.1186/s12894-015-0003-z

BMC
Urology

Transurethral cystolitholapaxy with the AH-1 stone removal system for the treatment of bladder stones of variable size

Aihua Li[1], Chengdong Ji[1], Hui Wang[1], Genqiang Lang[2*], Honghai Lu[1], Sikuan Liu[1], Weiwu Li[1], Binghui Zhang[1] and Wei Fang[1]

Abstract

Background: The treatment of large volume bladder stones by current equipments continues to be a management problem in both developing and developed countries. AH-1 Stone Removal System (SRS) invented by us is primarily used to crush and retrieve bladder stones. This study evaluated the safety and efficiency of transurethral cystolitholapaxy with SRS for the treatment of bladder stones of variable size.

Methods: SRS, which was invented by Aihua Li in 2007, composed by endoscope, continuous-flow component, a jaw for stone handling and retrieving, lithotripsy tube, handle, inner sheath and outer sheath. 112 patients with bladder stones were performed by transurethral cystolitholapaxy with SRS since 2008. We compare the surgical outcome to bladder stones of variable size, and evaluate the surgical efficiency and safety.

Results: Characteristics of patients and stone removal time in variable size were evaluated. To patients with single stone, stone size was 1.35 ± 0.37 cm and the operating time was 5.50 ± 3.92 min in Group A. Stone size was 2.38 ± 0.32 cm and the operating time was 11.90 ± 9.91 min in Group B. Stone size was 3.30 ± 0.29 cm and the operating time was 21.92 ± 9.44 min in Group C. Stone size was 4.69 ± 0.86 cm and the operating time was 49.29 ± 30.47 min in Group D. The difference was statistically significant between the four groups. Among them, 74 (66.07%) patients accompanied with benign prostatic hyperplasia (BPH) were treated by transurethral resection of the prostate (TURP) simultaneously. Compared between the four groups, the difference of the TURP time was not statistically significant, P >0.05. No significant complication was found in the surgical procedure.

Conclusions: Transurethral cystolitholapaxy with SRS appears to be increased rapidity of the procedure with decreased morbidity. It is a safe and efficient surgical management to bladder stones. This endoscopic surgery best fits the ethics principle of no injury; meanwhile, the accompanied BPH could be effectively treated by TURP simultaneously.

Keywords: Bladder stone, Transurethral cystolitholapaxy, Endoscopic surgery, AH-1 stone removal system

Background

Bladder stones account for 5% of urinary stones in the developed countries but for more in the developing countries. Novel modifications of these treatment modalities have been used for bladder stones. Unfortunately, the treatment of large volume bladder stones continues to be a management problem in both developing and developed countries [1-9].

Transurethral cystolitholapaxy is probably the most common way to manage cystolithiasis. But the transurethral methods by the current lithotriptoscope, nephroscope, cystoscope, resctoscope or ureteroscope are plagued by long operative times, trauma to the bladder mucosa, and still have several serious deficiencies [4,10-13]. SRS is primarily used to fragment and retrieve bladder stones, and is a dedicated endoscopic device with multiple functions such as stabilizing stone, fragmenting stone, automatically collecting fragments, retrieving stone, washing out stone and continuous irrigation in cystolitholapaxy. The primary

* Correspondence: zyhml103@sina.com
[2]Department of Urology, the 411th Hospital of PLA, Shanghai 200081, China
Full list of author information is available at the end of the article

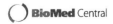

Li *et al. BMC Urology* (2015) 15:9

Page 2 of 5

outcome compared with a control group with current device appeared that the surgical procedure was safe and efficient [10-12].

The retrospective study was on 112 cases of bladder stones treated by transurethral cystolitholapaxy with SRS in last 7 years. We compare the surgical outcome to bladder stones of variable size, and further evaluate the surgical efficiency and safety.

Methods

Patients

Between July 2008 and March 2014, all 112 cases of bladder stone in our department were treated by transurethral cystolitholapaxy with SRS, after informed consents were obtained from patients. Among them, 74 (66.07%) patients accompanied with BPH were treated by TURP simultaneously. Follow-up was performed in 3 month postoperatively. Patients were between the ages of 43 and 97 years old, with a mean age of 74.1. Of these 112 patients, 97 were male and 15 were female.

112 patients were divided into four groups by the stone size. 54 patients with stone size <2 cm were in Group A, 34 patients with stone size from 2 to 2.9 cm were in Group B, 15 patients with stone size from 3 to 3.9 cm were in Group C, and 9 patients with stone size ≥4 cm were in Group D and the largest stone was 6.4 cm. The 54 patients in Group A were further divided to two subgroups by the surgical management to stones. Group A1 consisted of 10 patients and the stones were directly extracted using the jaw without lithotripsy; Group A2 had 44 patients and lithotripsy should be performed first and then fragments were retrieved. In 71 cases of bladder stone accompanied with BPH, TURP was performed with transurethral cystolitholapaxy simultaneously.

All patients were evaluated by physical examination, ultrasonography, plain abdominal radiography, complete blood count and blood biochemistry. The patients accompanied with BPH were further evaluated by International Prostate Symptom Score, serum prostate-specific antigen level. Stone size was measured by plain abdominal radiography and prostate volume was measured by ultrasonography or CT scan. The used irrigation fluid was saline in cystolitholapaxy and mannitol in TURP as usual.

Surgical instruments and techniques

These surgical procedures were performed in the lithotomy position under spinal anesthesia. Holmium laser was used to perform cystolithotripsy, and the power setting used of holmium laser was 2.6–3.5 J and 2.0–2.5 Hz. The procedures were as follows.

26 F SRS is composed by endoscope with illuminant and imaging component, continuous-flow component, a jaw for stone handling and stabilization during cystolithotripsy and stone retrieving during lithoextraction,

lithotripsy tube, handle, inner sheath and outer sheath (Figure 1). Inner diameter of the outer sheath is 8.2 mm and it can be connected with Ellik evacuator. Sphere >60 mm in diameter can be stabilized with the jaw, sphere <15 mm can be grasped directly, and sphere <8 mm can be retrieved through outer sheath. The lithotripsy tube is 1.4 mm in inner diameter, by which, holmium laser fiber or pneumatic lithotripter probe can be passed to perform cystolithotripsy. The entire device is usually attached to a video camera to provide vision for the surgeon [10-12].

During the surgical procedure, first the outer sheath with inner sheath and endoscope was introduced into bladder in visual and conventional cystoscopy could be performed to check and visualize stones (Figure 2). Then, the inner sheath was removed and the working component was inserted into the outer sheath. By improving design, the working component also can go through a standard resectoscope sheath by a connector. After entering bladder and visualizing stones, stones were grasped and fixed using the jaw, and then cystolithotripsy was performed with holmium laser through lithotripsy tube (Figure 3B). After lithotripsy is completed, fragments could be retrieved using the jaw through outer sheath synchronously (Figure 3C). If there were more residual smaller fragments, Ellik evacuator could be further connected with the outer sheath and fragments were retrieved by Ellik evacuator. To patients accompanied with BPH, resectoscope was reinserted into urethra to perform TURP after cystolitholapaxy. A standard 26 F continuous-flow Storz resectoscope with a wing loop was used. The electrosurgical generator (Bircher Type-4400, USA) was set to 280–290 W of pure cutting current for the incision and 80–90 W for coagulation. Prostate tissue was resected to the surgical capsule of the prostate during the operating procedure. All surgical procedures were performed by one surgeon. The patients without other diseases were discharged within 48 hours and the patients simultaneously performed TURP or bladder neck incision was discharged in 5-7 days postoperatively [10-12].

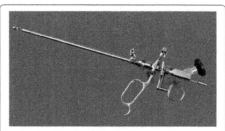

Figure 1 AH-1 stone removal system (SRS).

Li *et al. BMC Urology* (2015) 15:9

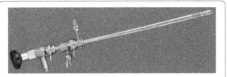

Figure 2 The outer sheath with inner sheath and endoscope.

SRS was designed by Aihua Li, M.D., and manufactured by Hangzhou Tonglu Shikonghou Medical Instrument Co., Ltd.

Ethical consent
The study was approved by the Medical Ethics Committee of Yangou Hospital, School of Medicine, Tongji University.

Statistical analysis
The differences of measurement data were compared using an unpaired t test and Chi-square test. Difference was considered significant at a P value <0.05. The reported values are the mean ± SD.

Results
In all the 15 (13.39%) female patients, 4 (7.40%) cases were in Group A, 4 (11.76%) cases in Group B, 3 (20.00%) cases in Group C and 4 (44.44%) cases in Group D. Group D was compared with Group A, the difference was statistically significant, P <0.05. Stone size, stone number, patients performed by TURP simultaneously and the prostate volume in the four groups are shown in Table 1.

In Group A1, stones were directly retrieved by the jaw through the outer sheath or through urethra outside the sheath without lithotripsy. In Group A2 and other three groups, cystolithotripsy should be performed first and then fragments were retrieved by the jaw. In the surgery, stones <0.7 cm can be easily retrieved by the jaw through the outer sheath and more fragments could be retrieved by one extracting procedure. Stone removal time in different stone sizes and patients with single stone are shown in Tables 2 and 3.

To 12 (10.71%) patients with BPH, the insertion of SRS was prevented by larger prostatic median lobe. So that TURP or bladder neck incision was first performed by F24 Storz resectoscope, to resect prostate or only the larger median lobe, and then cystolitholapaxy was performed. In this case, the surgical vision would be too blurred to perform surgery due to bleeding from resected fossa of prostate. In 4 (3.57%) patients with urethral stricture, urethral dilatation was performed first and then cystolithotripsy was done. But in another (0.89%) patients, the urethral stricture was too serious so that SRS was unable to be introduced into bladder. After

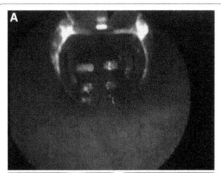

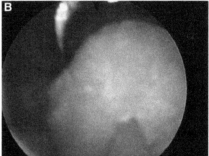

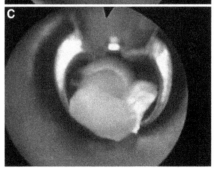

Figure 3 Characteristics and functions of the jaw. **A**. The jaw in endoscope; **B**. Stone was stabilized with the jaw and lithotripsy was performed with holmium laser; **C**. Fragments were retrieved using the jaw through outer sheath.

SRS was further improved, the equipment can be introduced into the bladder under direct vision. And then the difficulty inserting into bladder was markedly improved, it appeared only in 3 patients (6.98%) among the later 43 patients.

No other significant complication was found in the surgical procedure and no patient was converted to an

Li *et al. BMC Urology* (2015) 15:9

Table 1 Characteristics of patients

Group	N	Stone size (cm)	Stone number	BPH	Prostate volume (ml)
A1 (<2 cm)	10	0.84 ± 0.30	8.78 ± 8.45	9	44.87 ± 25.74
A2 (<2 cm)	44	1.43 ± 0.24	5.12 ± 6.36	31	56.93 ± 33.38
B (2-2.9 cm)	34	2.34 ± 0.31	2.62 ± 3.43	20	63.75 ± 42.71
C (3-3.9 cm)	15	3.27 ± 0.24	1.47 ± 1.20	10	63.12 ± 28.78
D (≥4 cm)	9	4.82 ± 0.83	2.44 ± 3.64	4	37.78 ± 18.04
Total	112			74	

Stone size was presented by the biggest in patients with multiple stones. Compared between the four groups, the difference of prostate volume was not statistically significant, P >0.05.

Table 3 Stone removal time of patients with single stone

Group	N	Stone size	Stone removal time (min)
A (<2 cm)	22	1.35 ± 0.37	5.50 ± 3.92
B (2-2.9 cm)	21	2.38 ± 0.32	11.90 ± 9.91
C (3-3.9 cm)	12	3.30 ± 0.29	21.92 ± 9.44
D (≥4 cm)	7	4.69 ± 0.86	49.29 ± 30.47

Compared with Group A, the difference of stone removal time was statistically significant, P <0.01 in Group B, P <0.001 in Group C and Group D. Compared with Group B, the difference was statistically significant, P <0.01 in Group C and P <0.001 in Group D. Compared with Group C, the difference was statistically significant, P <0.02 in Group D.

open procedure. The mean follow-up time was 35.18 ± 20.05 months (range 3-72 months) with no late complications related to the surgical procedure. None of the patients developed urethral stricture disease in the follow-up. All patients including whom with BPH and previously known urethral stricture disease had normal voiding function in the follow-up.

Discussion

In the last decades, variable techniques for management of bladder stones have been mentioned in literature [1-12]. Open cystolithotomy, extracorporeal shockwave lithotripsy, percutaneous cystolitholapaxy and transurethral cystolitholapaxy are commonly performed in different medical center. The classical treatment for bladder stones still is transurethral cystolitholapaxy with lithotriptoscope, nephroscope, cystoscope, resctoscope or ureteroscope [1,2,4,10-14]. But the transurethral methods are either time consuming or have high morbidity, because four major deficiencies still can't be perfectly resolved in the procedures [2]. First, bladder stone is easily rolling within bladder for the large cavity, which makes lithotripsy more difficult, especially to large volume or hard stone; Second, excessive fragments are produced after large bladder stone is

crushed, and men urethra is slender and curl so that lithoextraction is not easy; Third, bladder wall is too thin to be easily damaged and ruptured in filling condition by irrigating solution [3,4]. Moreover, the current forceps used in endoscopic surgery can't be used to stabilize stone during lithotripsy, only can be used to retrieve smaller stone and extract one fragment by one extracting procedure during lithoextraction [15]. Therefore, multiple entries to the urethra for lithoextraction would be needed, which will lead to urethral injury.

Bladder stones are rare in women [16,17]. In the study, patients with bladder stones in men were more than that in women and approximately 14% of all bladder stones occur in women, but with the stone size increasing, the proportion in women will be increased significantly.

In the surgical procedure, stones are stabilized with the jaw so that stones are no longer rolling in bladder, which makes lithotripsy more effective. Stones or fragments <7 mm can be easily retrieved by the jaw through the outer sheath. It effectively prevents multiple entries to the urethra and hence avoids possible urethral injury. The stones in 0.7-0.9 cm can be directly retrieved through urethra outside the sheath without lithotripsy, but the management will bring more injury to urethra so that it shouldn't be used repeatedly. For retrieving smaller residual fragments, it's also possible the use of a resectoscope connected to Ellik evacuator in order to avoid multiple entries to the urethra [10-12].

In the study, along with the increase of stone size, operating time is obviously increased. In 16 patients with BPH or urethral stricture, SRS was failure to be introduced into bladder, which was overcome by urethral dilatation, incision of the elevated bladder neck and TURP. Fortunately, after the structure of SRS was improved and the equipment can be introduced into the bladder under direct vision, the difficulty in insertion into the bladder was markedly improved [10-12].

About 15% patients were accompanied with bladder stones in the patients underwent TURP in our department. The surgical procedure can be safely combined with TURP [18-21]. We prefer to perform cystolitholapaxy first in the surgery, because surgical vision would

Table 2 Stone removal time in different stone sizes

Group	Lithotripsy	Stone removal time (min)	TURP time (min)
A1 (<2 cm)	No	5.10 ± 2.13	32.50 ± 14.10
A2 (<2 cm)	Yes	11.11 ± 11.96	35.97 ± 14.92
B (2-2.9 cm)	Yes	17.30 ± 14.36	35.20 ± 10.74
C (3-3.9 cm)	Yes	20.68 ± 9.04	31.70 ± 12.44
D (≥4 cm)	Yes	64.11 ± 40.14	25.00 ± 12.25

Compared with Group A1, the difference of stone removal time was statistically significant, P <0.05 in Group B, P <0.001 in Group C and Group D. Compared with Group A2, the difference of stone removal time was statistically significant, P <0.01 in Group B and Group C, and P <0.001 in Group D. Compared with Group B, the difference of stone removal time was statistically significant, P <0.001 in Group D. Compared with Group C, the difference of stone removal time was statistically significant, P <0.01 in Group D. Compared between the four groups, the difference of TURP operating time was not statistically significant, P >0.05.

Li *et al. BMC Urology* (2015) 15:9

be blurred after TURP, for associated bleeding from the resected fossa.

In the surgical procedure, working component should be introduced into bladder through the sheath in visual to avoid injury to urethra and bladder, after the sheath is inserted. Keeping low-pressure continuous irrigation and drainage to bladder during the surgical procedure is important to keep surgical vision clear and prevent bladder damage and rupture. For advanced aged and high risk patient, or too many, large and hard stones, the surgery could be performed in phases for surgical safety [10-12].

Conclusions

Transurethral cystitholapaxy by SRS appears to be increased rapidity of the procedure with decreased morbidity and is a safe and efficient surgery to bladder stones. The benefits of SRS apparently are the ability to grasp the stone to prevent moving whilst energy is being delivered to the stone and more rapid evacuation of crushed fragments. It also prevents multiple entries to the urethra and hence avoids possible urethral injury. It would be the better alternative for urologist to treat bladder stones. To the patients with urethral stricture and children, SRS in smaller size is needed to develop in the future [22,23].

Abbreviations
BPH: Benign prostatic hyperplasia; SRS: AH-1 stone removal system; TURP: Transurethral resection of the prostate.

Competing interests
The authors declare that they have no competing interests.

Authors' contributions
AL and HW contributed equally to this paper. AL and HW performed data collection and analysis, and drafted the manuscript. AL, CJ, HW, GL, HL, SL, WL, BZ and WF performed the operations. All authors have read and approved the final manuscript.

Acknowledgements
The study is financially supported by The Project to Popularize Advanced and Suitable Technology in Shanghai Public Health System (No. 2013SY063), which sponsored by Shanghai Municipal Commission of Health and Family Planning.
SRS could be purchased by Hangzhou Tonglu Shikonghou Medical Instrument Co., Ltd. China. Email: shikonghou@163.com, xushengyuan010@163.com. Tel. 0086-571-69966018.

Author details
¹Department of Urology, Yangpu Hospital, School of Medicine, Tongji University, 450 Tengyue Road, Shanghai 200090, China. ²Department of Urology, the 411th Hospital of PLA, Shanghai 200081, China.

Received: 17 September 2014 Accepted: 3 February 2015
Published online: 21 February 2015

References

1. Zhao J, Shi L, Gao Z, Liu Q, Wang K, Zhang P. Minimally invasive surgery for patients with bulky bladder stones and large benign prostatic hyperplasia simultaneously: a novel design. Urol Int. 2013;91:31–7.
2. Tan YK, Gupta DM, Weinberg A, Matteis AJ, Kotwal S, Gupta M. Minimally invasive percutaneous management of large bladder stones with a laparoscopic entrapment bag. J Endourol. 2014;28:61–4.
3. Kawahara T, Ito H, Terao H, Ogawa T, Uemura H, Kubota Y, et al. Stone area and volume are correlated with operative time for cystolithotripsy for bladder calculi using a holmium: yttrium garnet laser. Scand J Urol Nephrol. 2012;46:298–303.
4. Singh KJ, Kaur J. Comparison of three different endoscopic techniques in management of bladder calculi. Indian J Urol. 2011;27:10–3.
5. Torricelli FC, Mazzucchi E, Danilovic A, Coelho RF, Srougi M. Surgical management of bladder stones: literature review. Rev Col Bras Cir. 2013;40:227–33.
6. Dhabalia JV, Jain N, Kumar V, Nelivigi GG. Modified technique of percutaneous cystolithotripsy using a new instrument combined single-step trocar-dilator with self-retaining adjustable access sheath. Urology. 2011;77:1304–7.
7. Elbahnasy AM, Farhat YA, Aboramadan AR, Taha MR. Percutaneous cystolithotripsy using self-retaining laparoscopic trocar for management of large bladder stones. J Endourol. 2010;24:2037–41.
8. Elcioglu O, Ozden H, Guven G, Kabay S. Urinary bladder stone extraction and instruments compared in textbooks of Abul-Qasim Khalaf Ibn Abbas Alzahrawi (Albucasis) (930–1013) and Serefeddin Sabuncuoglu (1385–1470). J Endourol. 2010;24:1463–8.
9. Toktas G, Sacak V, Erkan E, Kocaaslan R, Demiray M, Unluer E, et al. Novel technique of cytolithotripsy for large bladder stones. Asian J Endosc Surg. 2013;6:245–8.
10. Li A, Lu H, Ji C, Liu S, Zhang F, Qian X, et al. Transurethral cystolithotripsy with a novel special endoscope. Urol Res. 2012;40:769–73.
11. Li A, Lu H, Liu S, Zhang Z, Qian X, Wang H, et al. A Novel Endoscope to Treat Bladder Stone. J Endourol Part B, Videourology 2011, 25(2):doi:10.1089
12. Liu S, Li A, Ji C, Lu H, Zhang F, Qian X, et al. Efficiency of Transurethral Cystolithotripsy with AH-1 stone removal system. J Mod Urol. 2013;18:437–40.
13. Philippou P, Volanis D, Kariotis I, Serafetinidis E, Delakas D. Prospective comparative study of endoscopic management of bladder lithiasis: is prostate surgery a necessary adjunct? Urology. 2011;78:43–7.
14. Tefekli A, Cezayirli F. The history of urinary stones: in parallel with civilization. Sci World J. 2013;2013:423964.
15. Ener K, Agras K, Aldemir M, Okulu E, Kayigil O. The randomized comparison of two different endoscopic techniques in the management of large bladder stones: transurethral use of nephroscope or cystoscope? J Endourol. 2009;23:1151–5.
16. Stav K, Dwyer PL. Urinary bladder stones in women. Obstet Gynecol Surv. 2012;67:715–25.
17. Hudson CO, Sinno AK, Northington GM, Galloway NT, Karp DR. Complete transvaginal surgical management of multiple bladder calculi and obstructed uterine procidentia. Female Pelvic Med Reconstr Surg. 2014;20:59–61.
18. Li A, Lu H, Liu S, Zhang F, Qian X, Wang H. Effect of Ageing on the Efficiency of TUVRP. The Aging Male. 2012;15:263–6.
19. Li A, Zhang Y, Lu H, Zhang F, Liu S, Wang H, et al. Living Status in Patients over 85 Years of Age after TUVRP. The Aging Male. 2013;16:191–4.
20. Speakman MJ, Cheng X. Management of the complications of BPH/BOO. Indian J Urol. 2014;30:208–13.
21. Childs MA, Mynderse LA, Rangel LJ, Wilson TM, Lingeman JE, Krambeck AE. Pathogenesis of bladder calculi in the presence of urinary stasis. J Urol. 2013;189:1347–51.
22. Ahmadnia H, Kamalati A, Younesi M, Imani MM, Moradi M, Esmaeili M. Percutaneous treatment of bladder stones in children: 10 years experience, is blind access safe? Pediatr Surg Int. 2013;29:725–8.
23. Uygun I, Okur MH, Aydogdu B, Arayici Y, Isler B, Otcu S. Efficacy and safety of endoscopic laser lithotripsy for urinary stone treatment in children. Urol Res. 2012;40:751–5.

Urol Res (2012) 40:769–773
DOI 10.1007/s00240-012-0503-1

ORIGINAL PAPER

Transurethral cystolithotripsy with a novel special endoscope

Aihua Li · Honghai Lu · Chengdong Ji · Sikuan Liu ·
Feng Zhang · Xiaoqiang Qian · Hui Wang

Received: 24 February 2012 / Accepted: 2 August 2012 / Published online: 26 August 2012
© Springer-Verlag 2012

Abstract To evaluate the safety and efficiency of the Aihua (AH)-1 stone removal system (SRS) to treat bladder stones. Thirty five patients with of bladder stones >2 cm and with benign prostatic hyperplasia were treated by transurethral cystolithotripsy with the SRS and TURP. The results in these patients were compared with 14 patients treated with current devices. In the SRS group, 26 patients had a single stone. Average stone size was 3.34 ± 1.03 cm, total operating time was 55.12 ± 19.95 min, and stone removal time was 23.30 ± 17.08 min. In the control group, 12 patients had a single stone. The average stone size was 2.46 ± 0.45 cm (larger stone size in SRS group, $P < 0.05$), total operating time was 79.85 ± 24.63 min (shorter operating time in SRS group, $P < 0.05$) and stone removal time was 43.28 ± 24.18 min the control group (shorter removal time in SRS group, $P < 0.05$). Mean stone size was 2.37 ± 1.18 cm and mean time to remove one stone was 12.57 ± 12.99 min in the SRS group. Mean stone size was 2.40 ± 0.48 cm (no significant difference between groups, $P > 0.05$) and mean time to remove one stone was 33.23 ± 25.26 min in the control group (shorter time in the SRA group, $P < 0.001$). No significant complication was found in the SRS group. This study suggests that multiple functions of SRS can be expected in transurethral cystolithotripsy. It can be used to fix stones during lithotripsy, and automatically collect stones and extract more stones through the sheath at one time during lithoextraction, which can reduce surgical time and damage to the bladder and urethra. This surgical procedure appears to be safe and efficient, and operating indications for transurethral cystolithotripsy could be expanded with this surgical procedure.

Keywords Bladder stone · Transurethral cystolithotripsy · Endoscope · AH-1 stone removal system

A. Li (✉) · H. Lu · C. Ji · S. Liu · F. Zhang · X. Qian ·
H. Wang
Department of Urology, Yangpu Hospital, Yangpu Distric
Central Hospital of Shanghai, Tongji University,
450 Tengyue Road, Shanghai 200090, China
e-mail: li121288@yahoo.com.cn

H. Lu
e-mail: julietlhh@sina.com

C. Ji
e-mail: longjcd@yahoo.com.cn

S. Liu
e-mail: liusikuan@126.com

F. Zhang
e-mail: tongku7328@yahoo.com.cn

X. Qian
e-mail: qxqshh@sohu.com

H. Wang
e-mail: wh78518@yahoo.com.cn

Introduction

The management of bladder calculi has been developed in the recent decade, with the result that multiple management modalities are available [1–9]. Transurethral approaches for bladder calculi or cystolitholapaxy is probably the most common way to manage cystolithiasis, and especially appropriate if there are associated bladder outlet pathologies [9–14]. But current transurethral cystolithotripsy still has several deficiencies, such as the used devices can't be used to fix stone, continuously irrigate and efficaciously extract fragments in cystolitholapaxy. The surgical difficulty will be increased when the stones are >2 cm. Stone removal system (SRS) invented by us, which is primarily used to crush and evacuate bladder stone, is an special

770

Urol Res (2012) 40:769–773

endoscope with multiple functions such as fixing stone, crushing stone, automatically gathering stone, extracting stone, washing out stone, and continuous irrigation in cystolithotripsy. Unusually, the minimal invasive device can be used to automatically collect stone and more fragments can be extracted at one time.

In the present study, the safety and efficiency of transurethral cystolithotripsy with SRS to treat bladder stone >2 cm were retrospectively evaluated after compared with current devices.

Patients and methods

Between January 2008 and January 2012, 35 cases of bladder stone with benign prostatic hyperplasia (BPH) were treated by transurethral cystolithotripsy with SRS and TURP in our department, after informed consents were obtained from patients, and they were separated as SRS group. These were compared with retrospective cohort of 14 cases of bladder stone with BPH treated by transurethral cystolithotripsy with current devices and TURP as control group. Follow-up was performed in 3 month postoperatively. Patient age was 48–97 years, with a mean age of 76.94 years. Stone size and operating time were respectively compared between the two groups.

All patients were evaluated by physical examination, International Prostate Symptom Score, complete blood count, blood biochemistry, serum prostate-specific antigen level, ultrasonography, and plain abdominal radiography. Prostate volume was measured by ultrasonography or CT scan, and stone size was measured by plain abdominal radiography. The used irrigation fluid was saline in cystolithotripsy and mannitol in TURP as usual.

Surgical instruments and techniques

These procedures were performed in the lithotomy position under spinal anesthesia. Holmium laser was used to perform lithotripsy, and the power setting used of holmium laser was 2.6–3.5 J and 2.0–2.5 Hz. Surgical procedures in the two groups were as follows:

SRS group

26F SRS is composed by illuminant and imaging component, continuous-flow component, a jaw to grasp and extract stone, lithotripsy tube, handle, and sheath (Photo 1). Inner diameter of the sheath is 8.2 mm and it can be connected with Ellik evacuator. Sphere >60 mm in diameter can be fixed with jaw by occlusive force and downward pressure, sphere <15 mm can be grasped directly, and sphere <8 mm

can be extracted through sheath. The lithotripsy tube is 1.4 mm in inner diameter, by which, holmium laser fiber or pneumatic lithotripter probe can be transited to perform lithotripsy. The entire device is usually attached to a video camera to provide vision for the surgeon.

During the surgical procedure, first SRS was inserted into bladder to search stone. Then, stone was graspbed and fixed using jaw, and lithotripsy was performed with holmium laser through lithotripsy tube (Photo 2). Fragments could be extracted using jaw through sheath synchronously (Photo 3). If there were more smaller residual fragments, Ellik evacuator could be connected with sheath to wash out them. Finally, resectoscope was inserted in urethra to perform TURP.

The endoscope was designed by Aihua Li, M.D., and manufactured by Hangzhou Tonglu Shikonghou Medical Instrument Co., Ltd.

Control group

A 26F Storz continuous-flow resectoscope was used in the procedure. After resectoscope was inserted in urethra, stones were fixed with the sheath. Then, lithotripsy was performed by an 8F Storz ureteroscope using holmium laser through resectoscope sheath. Fragments were washed out with Ellik evacuator and larger residual fragments could be extracted using wire loop of resectoscope through urethra. TURP was performed immediately after above procedure.

The surgery in the two groups was performed by one surgeon.

Statistical analysis

The differences of measurement data were compared using an unpaired t test and Chi-square test. Difference was considered significant at a P value <0.05. The reported values are the mean ± SD.

Results

The characteristics and operative parameters in the two groups are shown in Tables 1, 2, 3.

Nine patients (25.71 %) were with multiple stones and a cumulative total of all stones was seventy in SRS group. Two patients (14.29 %) were with multiple stones and the total stone was seventeen in control group.

In control group, 3 cases (21.43 %) were converted to an open procedure, in which, 1 case for bladder perforation due to mucosal damage and 2 cases for excessive residual fragments to be removed. Furthermore, urethral stricture was developed in other 2 cases in 3 month postoperatively. In SRS group, TURP was performed first in three patients

Urol Res (2012) 40:769–773

Table 1 Characteristics of patients

	N	Age	Stone size (cm)	Prostate volume (ml)
SRS group	35	78.09 ± 5.17	3.30 ± 1.09 (2.0–6.4)	60.25 ± 39.58
Control group	14	74.07 ± 12.88	2.54 ± 0.46 (2.0–3.0)	52.16 ± 43.80

SRS group was compared with control group, the difference of stone size ($P < 0.05$) was statistically significant but the difference of age and prostate volume was not

Table 2 Operating time of patients with single stone

	SRS group	Control group
Case	26	12
Stone size (cm)	3.34 ± 1.03	2.46 ± 0.45
Total operating time (min)	55.12 ± 19.95	79.85 ± 24.63
TURP time (min)	31.82 ± 9.49	36.57 ± 11.82
Stone removal time (min)	23.30 ± 17.08	43.28 ± 24.18

Compared between the two groups, the difference of stone size ($P < 0.05$), total operating time ($P < 0.05$) and stone removal time ($P < 0.05$) was statistically significant

Table 3 Mean time to remove one stone

	SRS group	Control group
Case	35	14
Total stone	70	17
Mean stone number	2.18	1.21
Biggest stone (cm)	6.4	3
Mean stone size (cm)	2.37 ± 1.18	2.40 ± 0.48
Mean time to remove one stone (min)	12.57 ± 12.99	33.23 ± 25.26

Compared between the two groups, the difference of mean time to remove one stone ($P < 0.001$) was statistically significant but the difference of mean stone size was not

for urethral stricture or larger median lobe of prostate. No significant complication was found in the surgical procedure. However, a patient with multiple stones who was 97 years old, with a largest stone in 5.8 cm, second lager stone in 2.2 cm and other 15 stones <2 cm, undergone a second endoscopic procedure at 14 day postoperatively for surgical safety. To other 2 case with severe urethral stricture, urethral dilatation was performed first, and then TURP was performed with a 24F Storz resectoscope, cystolithotripsy was successfully accomplished finally. But surgical vision was too blurred to perform due to bleeding from resected fossa of prostate.

Discussion

Variety of treatment modalities have been mentioned in literature regarding removal of bladder stone—open surgical, lithotripsy, percutaneous, and transurethral [1–8]. But the most commonly used contemporary treatment for bladder stones is transurethral cystolithotripsy [8–14]. It can be performed using lithotriptoscope, ureteroscope, nephroscope, cystoscope and resectoscope. But until now, three major deficiencies still can't be perfectly resolved in the procedures. First, bladder stone is easily rolling within bladder for the large cavity, which makes fragmentation more difficult sometimes, especially to larger stone; Second, excessive fragments are produced after large bladder stone is crushed, but men urethra is slender and curl so that lithoextraction is much hard; Finally, some current devices can't be continuously irrigated so that surgical vision is poor in the procedure, which makes bladder mucosa easily injured. It even leads to bladder perforation, especially when bladder is filled by irrigating solution.

Nephroscope has distinct advantage over other current endoscopes in transurethral cystolithotripsy as it has a wider lumen, which facilitates easy removal of the stone fragments. But current forceps only can be used to extract smaller stone, remove one fragment at one time and can't be used to fix stone during lithotripsy [9]. Meanwhile, repeated lithoextraction through urethra would be damage to urothelium.

Resectoscope sheath could be used to fix stone and then lithotripsy is performed through the sheath by ureteroscope. Resectoscope could be connected with Ellik evacuator and smaller fragments can be washed out through working tunnel. In the surgery, larger fragments could be extracted using wire loop through urethra but the electrode sheathed is made by wire so that it is easily damaged and the fixer to wire loop would be damaged after reiterative application in such way. Furthermore, the efficiency to fix stone is obviously not good as the jaw of SRS and will be sharply decreased when stone size is >2 cm. Therefore, this method is more applicable to bladder stone <2 cm.

In the study, the designed multiple functions of SRS had been shown in cystolitholapaxy. The jaw, like a ring in longitudinal, is located at the front of objective lens and open downward, and the central part still is a circular cavity when it is closed. The lithotripsy tube is located at the lower edge of objective lens, which facilitates fragmentation in direct vision. Two jaw pieces are frame-shaped, which is favorable to grasp and fix stone. Two little

Urol Res (2012) 40:769–773

Fig. 1 The principle of swing flow

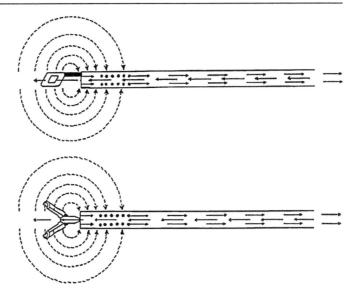

bars are installed at the far end of jaw so that it can be used to extract stone fragments through sheath as a trawler and more fragments can be extracted at one time. On other hand, Ellik evacuator can be connected with sheath to wash out smaller fragments. The principle of swing flow is applied in design, which makes the device to collect fragments automatically (Fig. 1). In stone fragmentation, holmium laser fiber or pneumatic lithotripter probe can be transited through lithotripsy tube to crush stones.

In the surgical procedure, stones are fixed with jaw and then are crushed, which makes fragmentation more effective for that stones are no longer rolling in bladder. Fragments <8 mm can be extracted with jaw through sheath or washed out using Ellik evacuator. As a result, the sheath doesn't have to be repeatedly inserted through urethra and which will effectively reduce damage to urethral mucosa. In some instances, larger fragments could be extracted through urethra, but the management will bring more injury to urethra so that it shouldn't be used repeatedly.

In the surgical procedure, to avoid injury to urethra and bladder, after sheath of SRS is inserted, working component should be inserted into bladder through the sheath always in direct vision. Frequent drainage of the bladder or low-pressure continuous irrigation during the procedure is important to prevent bladder rupture. Keeping continuous irrigation in procedure is of great benefit to keeping surgical vision clear and preventing bladder damage. For advanced aged and high risk patient, or too many, large and hard stones, surgery could be performed in phases. We prefer to remove bladder stone first in surgery of SRS combined with TURP, because surgical vision may not be as clear after TURP, for associated hematuria from the resected fossa. However, if median lobe of prostate is too large to perform fragmentation, the median lobe could be resected first in order to facilitate operation.

Transurethral lithotripsy can be safely combined with TURP, with one study showing slightly higher complication rate from hematuria when compared with TURP alone [11–14]. Combined TURP and percutaneous cystolithotripsy is safer, more effective, and much faster alternative to combined TURP and transurethral cystolithotripsy in patients with large bladder stones and BPH [2–4, 15]. In principle, SRS also can be used in percutaneous procedure. But in the study, the largest stone in SRS group was 6.40 cm and it was successfully crushed and extracted through urethra using the device so that bladder puncture has been satisfyingly avoided.

Conclusions

Our study shows that multiple functions such as fixing stone, crushing stone, automatically gathering stone, extracting stone, washing out stone and continuous irrigation can be expected when SRS is applied in transurethral cystolithotripsy. Especially, it can be used to fix stones

 Springer

Urol Res (2012) 40:769–773

during lithotripsy, and automatically collect stone and extract more stones through sheath at one time during lithoextraction, which can effectively reduce stone removal time and surgical damage to bladder and urethra. This minimally invasive endoscopic procedure appears to be safe and efficient, which could expand the operating indication on transurethral cystolithotripsy. Additional randomized trials comparing other endoscopes are warranted to delineate the best device to manage bladder stone.

Conflict of interest No competing financial interests exist.

References

1. Wong M (2008) Bladder calculi, an evidence-based review. In: Stone disease. The 2nd international consultation on stone disease. Editions 21, Paris, pp 295–303
2. Dhabalia JV, Jain N, Kumar V, Nelivigi GG (2011) Modified technique of percutaneous cystolithotripsy using a new instrument–combined single-step trocar-dilator with self-retaining adjustable access sheath. Urology 77(6):1304–1307
3. Tugcu V, Polat H, Ozbay B, Gurbuz N, Eren GA, Tasci AI (2009) Percutaneous versus transurethral cystolithotripsy. J Endourol 23(2):237–241
4. Elbahnasy AM, Farhat YA, Aboramadan AR, Taha MR (2010) Percutaneous cystolithotripsy using self-retaining laparoscopic trocar for management of large bladder stones. J Endourol 24(12):2037–2041
5. Al-Marhoon MS, Sarhan OM, Awad BA, Helmy T, Ghali A, Dawaba MS (2009) Comparison of endourological and open cystolithotomy in the management of bladder stones in children. J Urol 181(6):2684–2687 (discussion 2687–2688)
6. Lam PN, Te CC, Wong C, Kropp BP (2007) Percutaneous cystolithotomy of large urinary-diversion calculi using a combination of laparoscopic and endourologic techniques. J Endourol 21:155–157
7. Elcioglu O, Ozden H, Guven G, Kabay S (2010) Urinary bladder stone extraction and instruments compared in textbooks of Abul-Qasim Khalaf Ibn Abbas Alzahrawi (Albucasis) (930–1013) and Serefeddin Sabuncuoglu (1385–1470). J Endourol 24(9):1463–1468
8. Singh KJ, Kaur J (2011) Comparison of three different endoscopic techniques in management of bladder calculi. Indian J Urol 27(1):10–13
9. Ener K, Agras K, Aldemir M, Okulu E, Kayigil O (2009) The randomized comparison of two different endoscopic techniques in the management of large bladder stones: transurethral use of nephroscope or cystoscope? J Endourol 23(7):1151–1155
10. Kara C, Resorlu B, Cicekbilek I, Unsal A (2009) Transurethral cystolithotripsy with holmium laser under local anesthesia in selected patients. Urology 74(5):1000–1003
11. Philippou P, Volanis D, Kariotis I, Serafetinidis E, Delakas D (2011) Prospective comparative study of endoscopic management of bladder lithiasis: is prostate surgery a necessary adjunct? Urology 78(1):43–47
12. Shah HN, Hegde SS, Shah JN, Mahajan AP, Bansal MB (2007) Simultaneous transurethral cystolithotripsy with holmium laser enucleation of the prostate: a prospective feasibility study and review of literature. BJU Int 99(3):595–600
13. Aron M, Goel R, Gautam G, Seth A, Gupta NP (2007) Percutaneous versus transurethral cystolithotripsy and TURP for large prostates and large vesical calculi: refinement of technique and updated data. Int Urol Nephrol 39(1):173–177
14. Kamat NK (2003) Transurethral resection of prostate and suprapubic ballistic vesicolithotrity for benign prostatic hyperplasia with vesical calculi. J Endourol 17(7):505–509
15. Demirel F, Cakan M, Yalcinkaya F et al (2006) Percutaneous superaoubic cystolithotripsy approach: for whom? Why? J Endourol 20:429–431

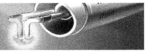

PlasmaButton™ Vaporization Therapy in Saline

Home　Publications　Resources　Librarians　Press　Advertise

Liebert Connect　　MY LIEBERT

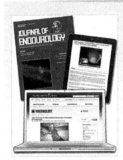

Read Online ▸　　Subscribe/Renew ▸　　For Authors ▸

Journal of Endourology and Part B, Videourology

Co-Editors-in-Chief: Ralph V. Clayman and Arthur D. Smith

ISSN: 0892-7790 • Published Monthly • Online ISSN: 1557-900X

Current Volume: 27

Latest Impact Factor* is 2.074

*2012 Journal Citation Reports® published by Thomson Reuters, 2013

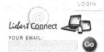

VIDEOUROLOGY™
Submit your videos today!

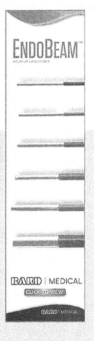

ENDOBEAM™

Featured Press Releases and Editorial Content

- WCE 2012 Istanbul Abstracts Now Online...Read Now
- 2011 Translated Abstracts (Chinese, Japanese, German, Polish, Russian, Turkish)...Read Now
- 20th Anniversary of First Laparoscopic Nephrectomy Celebrated in *Journal of Endourology* (Read More)...and corresponding videos in *Videourology* (Read More)
- Groundbreaking *Videourology* Journal Launched by Mary Ann Liebert, Inc....Let's See It

OVERVIEW

The leading journal of minimally invasive urology for over 25 years, *Journal of Endourology* is the essential publication for practicing surgeons who want to keep up with the latest surgical technologies in endoscopic, laparoscopic, robotic, and image-guided procedures as they apply to benign and malignant diseases of the genitourinary tract. This flagship journal includes the companion videojournal *Videourology*™ with every subscription. While *Journal of Endourology* remains focused on publishing rigorously peer reviewed articles, *Videourology* accepts original videos containing material that has not been reported elsewhere, except in the form of an abstract or a conference presentation.

Journal of Endourology coverage includes:

- The latest laparoscopic, robotic, endoscopic, and image-guided techniques for treating both benign and malignant conditions
- Pioneering research articles
- Controversial cases in endourology
- Techniques in endourology with accompanying videos
- Reviews and epochs in endourology
- Endourology survey section of endourology relevant manuscripts published in other journals

About This Publication:

Overview
Editorial Board
Manuscript Submission
Read Online/TOC
Press Releases
Testimonials
Featured Content
Subscribe/Renew
Recommend this title to your Library or Institution
Reprints, Rights, & Permissions
Advertising
Fast Facts
Multi-site Licenses
Disclaimer

Download a screensaver ▸

Sample Content ▸

• OPEN Access : Options & Benefits

BARD | MEDICAL

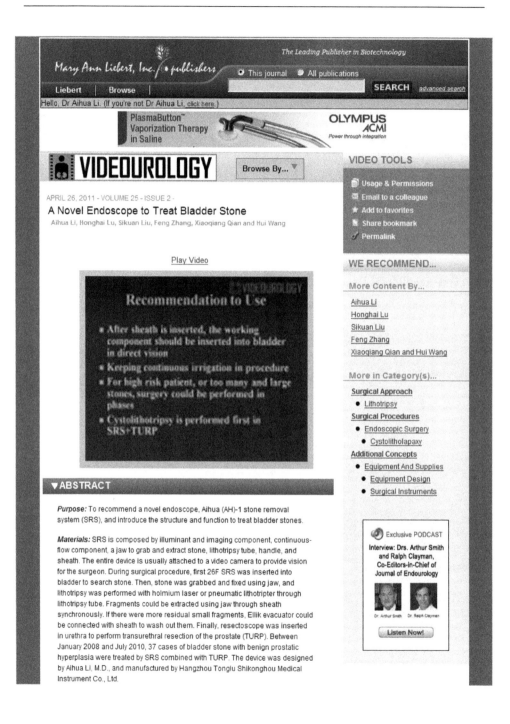

The Leading Publisher in Biotechnology

Mary Ann Liebert, Inc. / publishers

○ This journal   ○ All publications

SEARCH   advanced search

Liebert | Browse

Hello, Dr Aihua Li. (If you're not Dr Aihua Li, click here.)

PlasmaButton™
Vaporization Therapy
in Saline

OLYMPUS
ACMI
Power through integration

VIDEOUROLOGY

Browse By... ▼

VIDEO TOOLS

- Usage & Permissions
- Email to a colleague
- Add to favorites
- Share bookmark
- Permalink

APRIL 26, 2011 - VOLUME 25 - ISSUE 2 -

A Novel Endoscope to Treat Bladder Stone

Aihua Li, Honghai Lu, Sikuan Liu, Feng Zhang, Xiaoqiang Qian and Hui Wang

Play Video

Recommendation to Use

- After sheath is inserted, the working component should be inserted into bladder in direct vision
- Keeping continuous irrigation in procedure
- For high risk patient, or too many and large stones, surgery could be performed in phases
- Cystolithotripsy is performed first in SRS+TURP

WE RECOMMEND...

More Content By...

Aihua Li
Honghai Lu
Sikuan Liu
Feng Zhang
Xiaoqiang Qian and Hui Wang

More in Category(s)...

Surgical Approach
- Lithotripsy

Surgical Procedures
- Endoscopic Surgery
  - Cystolitholapaxy

Additional Concepts
- Equipment And Supplies
- Equipment Design
- Surgical Instruments

Exclusive PODCAST

Interview: Drs. Arthur Smith and Ralph Clayman, Co-Editors-in-Chief of Journal of Endourology

Dr. Arthur Smith   Dr. Ralph Clayman

Listen Now!

▼ABSTRACT

Purpose: To recommend a novel endoscope, Aihua (AH)-1 stone removal system (SRS), and introduce the structure and function to treat bladder stones.

Materials: SRS is composed by illuminant and imaging component, continuous-flow component, a jaw to grab and extract stone, lithotripsy tube, handle, and sheath. The entire device is usually attached to a video camera to provide vision for the surgeon. During surgical procedure, first 26F SRS was inserted into bladder to search stone. Then, stone was grabbed and fixed using jaw, and lithotripsy was performed with holmium laser or pneumatic lithotripter through lithotripsy tube. Fragments could be extracted using jaw through sheath synchronously. If there were more residual small fragments, Ellik evacuator could be connected with sheath to wash out them. Finally, resectoscope was inserted in urethra to perform transurethral resection of the prostate (TURP). Between January 2008 and July 2010, 37 cases of bladder stone with benign prostatic hyperplasia were treated by SRS combined with TURP. The device was designed by Aihua Li, M.D., and manufactured by Hangzhou Tonglu Shikonghou Medical Instrument Co., Ltd.

Results: In the experiment *in vitro*, sphere >60 mm in diameter can be fixed with jaw by occlusive force and downward pressure, sphere <15 mm can be grabbed directly, and sphere <8 mm can be extracted through sheath. Inner diameter of the sheath is 8.2 mm, and it can be connected with Ellik evacuator. The lithotripsy tube is 1.4 mm in inner diameter, by which, holmium laser fiber or pneumatic lithotripter probe can be transited to perform lithotripsy. In the clinical study, the designed multiple functions had been showed in cystolithotripsy. The jaw, like a ring in longitudinal, is located at the front of objective lens and open downward, and the central part still is a circular cavity when it is closed. The lithotripsy tube is located at the lower edge of objective lens, which facilitates fragmentation in direct vision. Two jaw pieces are frame-shaped, which is favorable to grab and fix stone. Two little bars are installed at the far end of jaw so that it can be used to extract stone fragments through sheath as a trawler and more fragments can be extracted at one time. On other hand, Ellik evacuator can be connected with sheath to wash out small fragments. The principle of swing flow is applied in design that makes the device to collect fragments automatically. In stone fragmentation, holmium laser fiber or pneumatic lithotripter probe can be transited through lithotripsy tube to crush stones. Stones in 19 patients were <2 cm, the mean size was 1.36 ± 0.33 (0.7–1.8) cm, and stone removal time was 6.32 ± 4.44 min. Among these patients, those with multiple stones were five (35.71%), the stone number was 3.2 ± 1.30, and mean size was 1.24 ± 0.25 cm. Stones in other 18 patients were >2 cm, the mean size was 3.49 ± 1.32 (2.0–6.4) cm, and stone removal time was 32.88 ± 24.21 min. Among these patients, those with multiple stones were six (37.50%), the stone number was 6.67 ± 6.67, and mean size was 2.51 ± 0.93 cm. TURP was performed first in three patients for urethral stricture or larger median lobe of prostate. No significant complication was found in the surgical procedure. However, a patient with multiple stone who was 97 years old, with a largest stone in 5.8 cm, second lager stone in 2.2 cm, and other 15 stones <2 cm, undergone a second endoscopic procedure at 14 day postoperatively for surgical safety.

Conclusion: SRS is a novel endoscope with multiple functions to treat bladder stone. Our study shows that multiple functions such as fixing stone, crushing stone, automatically gathering stone, extracting stone, washing out stone, and continuous-flow can be expected when SRS is applied in cystolithotripsy. Especially, it can be used to automatically collect stone by swirling flow and extract more stones by jaw through sheath at one time, which can effectively reduce stone removal time and surgical damage to urethral mucosa. SRS combined with TURP is an effective and rapid modality to treat bladder stone with benign prostatic hyperplasia.[1–6] This minimally invasive endoscopic procedure appears to be safe and efficient, and could expand the range of operating indications on cystolithotripsy. Additional randomized trials comparing other endoscopes are warranted to delineate the best device to manage bladder stone.[7–11]

No competing financial interests exist.

Runtime of video: 9 mins 20 secs

▼CITE THIS VIDEO

Li A, Lu H, Liu S, Zhang F, Qian X, Wang H. A Novel Endoscope to Treat Bladder Stone. Journal of Endourology Part B, Videourology. March 2011, 25. doi: 10.1089/vid.2010.0090

▼REFERENCES

- 1. Wong M. Bladder calculi, an evidence-based review. In: Stone Disease. The 2nd International Consultation on Stone Disease. Paris: Editions 21, 2008, pp. 295–303.
- 2. Hammad FT, Kaya M, Kazim E. Bladder calculi: Did the clinical picture change? Urology 2006;67:1154–1158.
- 3. Li A, Lu H, Liu S, Zhang F, Qian X, Wang H. The clinical features of BPH in patients of advanced age and the efficiency of TUVRP. J Mod Urol 2009;14:291–294.
- 4. Ener K, Agras K, Aldemir M, Okulu E, Kayigil O. The randomized comparison of two different endoscopic techniques in the management of large bladder stones: Transurethral use of nephroscope or cystoscope? J Endourol 2009;23:1151–1157. [Abstract] [Medline]
- 5. Ringel RSA, Sluzker D. Combined cystolithotomy and transurethral resection of prostate: Best management of infravesical obstruction and massive or multiple bladder stones. Urology 2002;59:688–691.
- 6. Asci R, Aybek Z, Sarikaya S, Büyükalpelli R, Yilmaz AF. The management of vesical calculi with combined optical mechanical cystolithotripsy and transurethral prostatectomy: Is it safe and effective? BJU Int 1999;84:32–36. [CrossRef] [Medline]
- 7. Tugcu V, Polat H, Ozbay B, Gurbuz N, Eren GA, Tasci AI. Percutaneous versus transurethral cystolithotripsy. J Endourol 2009;23:237–241. [Abstract] [Medline]
- 8. Aron M, Goel R, Gautam G, Seth A, Gupta NP. Percutaneous versus transurethral cystolithotripsy and TURP for large prostates and large vesical calculi: Refinement of technique and updated data. Int Urol Nephrol 2007;39:173–177. [CrossRef] [Medline]
- 9. Demirel F, Cakan M, Yalcinkaya F, et al. Percutaneous superaoubic cystolithotripsy approach: For whom? Why? J Endourol 2006;20:429–431. [Abstract] [Medline]
- 10. Lam PN, Te CC, Wong C, Kropp BP. Percutaneous cystolithotomy of large urinary-diversion calculi using a combination of laparoscopic and endourologic techniques. J Endourol 2007;21:155–157. [Abstract] [Medline]
- 11. Al-Marhoon MS, Sarhan OM, Awad BA, Helmy T, Ghali A, Dawaba MS. Comparison of endourological and open cystolithotomy in the management of bladder stones in children. J Urol 2009;181:2684–2687. [CrossRef] [Medline]

AUTHOR INFORMATION

Li A, Department of Urology, Yangpu District Central Hospital, Shanghai, China. E-mail: li121288@yahoo.com.cn

Lu H, Department of Urology, Yangpu District Central Hospital, Shanghai, China.

Liu S, Department of Urology, Yangpu District Central Hospital, Shanghai, China.

Zhang F, Department of Urology, Yangpu District Central Hospital, Shanghai, China.

Qian X, Department of Urology, Yangpu District Central Hospital, Shanghai, China.

Wang H, Department of Urology, Yangpu District Central Hospital, Shanghai, China.

Mary Ann Liebert, Inc., publishers
140 Huguenot Street
New Rochelle, NY 10801-5215

现代泌尿外科杂志 2013年9月第18卷第5期 437

·论 著·

文章编号:1009-8291(2013)05-0437-04

AH-1型取石系统经尿道膀胱碎石的疗效评估

刘思宽,李爱华,嵇承栋,陆鸿海,张 峰,钱小强,王 珲,方 炜,张炳辉

(同济大学附属杨浦医院,上海市杨浦区中心医院泌尿外科,上海 200090)

Efficacy of transurethral cystolithotripsy with AH-1 stone removal system

LIU Si-kuan, LI Ai-hua, JI Cheng-dong, LU Hong-hai, ZHANG Feng, QIAN Xiao-qiang, WANG Hui, FANG Wei, ZHANG Bing-hui

(Department of Urology, Yangpu Hospital, School of Medicine, Tongji University, Shanghai 200090, China)

ABSTRACT:Objective To evaluate the safety and efficacy of Aihua (AH)-1 stone removal system (SRS) to treat bladder stones. Methods Data of 74 patients with bladder stone and benign prostatic hyperplasia (BPH) treated by transurethral cystolithotripsy with SRS and transurethral resection of prostate (TURP) were retrospectively compared with data of 50 patients treated with transurethral ureteroscopic lithotripsy and TRUP. The 74 patients were taken as the SRS group and the 50 patients the control group. Results In the SRS group, the diameters of stone size <2 cm were greater than the diameter of stone size in the control group. The differences of total operating time ($P<0.02$) and stone removal time ($P<0.001$) were statistically significant in patients with stone size <2 cm. The difference of total operating time and stone removal time were statistically significant in patients with single stone size $\geqslant2$ cm ($P<0.05$). The differences of mean time to remove one stone were statistically significant in patients with stone $\geqslant2$ cm ($P<0.001$). No significant complication was found in SRS group. Conclusions
Multiple functions of SRS can be expected in transurethral cystolithotripsy. It can be used to fix stones during lithotripsy, and automatically collect stones and extract more stones through the sheath at one time during lithoextraction, which can reduce operation time and damage to the bladder and urethra. This surgical procedure appears to be safe and effective, and operating indications for transurethral cystolithotripsy could be expanded with this surgical procedure.

KEY WORDS:bladder stone; transurethral cystolithotripsy; endoscope; AH-1 stone removal system

摘要:目的 评估AH-1型取石系统(SRS系统)治疗膀胱结石的安全性和疗效。方法 采用SRS系统经尿道碎石+经尿道前列腺电切术(TURP)治疗的膀胱结石伴前列腺增生(BPH)74例结石患者,与经尿道输尿管镜碎石+TURP治疗的50例结石患者的临床资料进行回顾性比较。直径<2 cm和≥2 cm结石分别评估。结果 SRS组<2 cm结石直径大于对照组(P<0.001)。二组相比,<2 cm结石患者的总手术时间和结石清除时间均少于对照组(P<0.02,P<0.001),单发性≥2 cm结石患者的总手术时间和结石清除时间差异有显著性(P<0.05)。≥2 cm结石组清除一枚结石所需平均手术时间差异有统计学意义(P<0.001)。SRS系统组无严重并发症发生。结论 SRS系统可提供固定结石、提供碎石通道、自动收集碎石、摄取碎石、冲吸碎石和连续冲洗等功能。尤其是可固定结石、自动收集碎石、一次可摄取多枚碎石。这样可缩短手术时间,拓展内镜治疗膀胱结石的手术适应范围。其联合TURP用于治疗膀胱结石伴BPH是一种安全、有效的治疗方法。

关键词:膀胱结石;经尿道碎石;内镜;AH-1型取石系统

中图分类号:R694.4 文献标志码:A

近10年来膀胱结石的治疗方法得到不断改进,经尿道碎石已经成为最主要的方法[1-9]。但是目前不同的经尿道膀胱碎石术依然存在一些重大缺陷,术中

收稿日期:2013-01-15 修回日期:2013-05-25
基金项目:2012年上海市杨浦区人才发展专项资金(鼎元资金)高层次人才科研成果转化类资金(No.201208)
通讯作者:李爱华,主任医师,E-mail:lii21288@yahoo.com.cn
作者简介:刘思宽(1970-),学士学位,主治医师.研究方向:腔内微创技术的临床应用和基础研究.E-mail:liusikuan@126.com

无法固定结石,不能进行持续冲洗、碎石取出较困难,当结石直径>2 cm时手术难度将明显增加。为了解决上述缺陷,我们研制了AH-1型取石系统(Aihua-1 stone removal system,SRS)系统,其具有固定结石、提供碎石通道、自动收集碎石、冲吸碎石、摄取碎石和连续冲洗等功能[10-11]。本文对照常用的输尿管镜联合电切镜膀胱碎石术,回顾性探讨SRS系统治疗膀胱结石的安全性和疗效,现报告如下。

1 材料与方法

1.1 临床资料 我院 2008 年 1 月至 2012 年 12 月年共采用 SRS 系统联合经尿道前列腺电切术（transurethral resection of prostate, TURP）一期治疗治疗膀胱结石伴前列腺增生（benign prostatic hyperplasia, BPH）74 例，年龄 74.3 岁。对照组输尿管镜碎石联合经尿道前列腺电切术 TURP 治疗膀胱结石伴 BPH 50 例，年龄 73.2 岁。直径＜2 cm 和≥2 cm 结石分别进行评估，≥2 cm 结石组最大结石直径均≥2 cm，统计结石数目时包含所有≥1 cm 结石。

1.2 手术器械和方法 各组均在脊柱麻醉下取截石位，钬激光碎石所用功率为 2.6～3.5 J 和 2.0～2.5 Hz。

1.2.1 SRS 组[10-11] F26 SRS 系统由窥镜光源成像系统、手柄、取石钳、碎石通道、液体连续冲洗系统、镜桥、镜鞘等部件组成（图 1）。可用取石钳夹固定直径＞6 cm 的球体。镜鞘内径 8.2 mm，可与 Ellick 冲吸器连接。镜鞘内可摄取直径＜0.8 cm 球体，镜鞘外可摄取直径＜1.5 cm 球体。碎石通道内径 1.4 mm，可通过气压弹道碎石杆或钬激光光纤。术中可通过镜桥直视下经尿道置入 SRS 系统，然后更换取石钳，寻及结石后固定结石。应用钬激光粉碎结石，

再用取石钳或 Ellick 冲吸器取出碎石，然后行 TURP。

SRS 系统由李爱华发明设计，杭州桐庐时空候医疗器械有限公司生产。

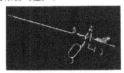

图 1　AH-1 型取石系统实物照片

1.2.2 对照组[3] 经尿道置入 F26 连续冲洗型 Storze 电切镜，寻及结石后用镜鞘固定。镜鞘内置入 F8 Storze 输尿管镜，钬激光碎石后再行 TURP。

1.3 统计学方法 对数据资料均以 $\bar{x} \pm s$ 表示，采用两独立样本的 t 检验进行差异显著性检验。假设检验的显著性水准取 $\alpha = 0.05$。

2 结　果

2.1 两组患者的临床基本资料 SRS 组＜2 cm 结石的直径大于对照组，差异有统计学意义（$P<0.001$），二组间≥2 cm 结石直径、年龄及前列腺体积差异无统计学意义（$P>0.05$，表 1）。

表 1　两组患者临床资料 ($\bar{x}\pm s$)

组别	例数	结石直径＜2 cm			例数	结石直径≥2 cm		
		年龄（岁）	结石直径（cm）	前列腺体积（mL）		年龄（岁）	结石直径（cm）	前列腺体积（mL）
SRS 组	30	70.66±10.19	1.39±0.31	42.09±23.63	44	76.48±8.76	3.11±1.06	56.44±38.20
对照组	36	70.26±10.13	0.98±0.40	51.18±27.81	14	74.07±12.88	2.54±0.46	52.16±43.80
t 值		1.025 6	4.562 6	1.113 8		0.795 2	1.947 7	0.320 8
P 值		＞0.05	＜0.001	＞0.05		＞0.05	＞0.05	＞0.05

2.2 两组患者的手术情况 二组相比，＜2 cm 结石及单发性≥2 cm 结石的总手术时间和结石清除时间 SRS 组均少于对照组，差异有统计学意义（$P<0.05$，表 2）。

在＜2 cm 结石中 SRS 组 15 例（50.00%）为多发性结石，对照组为 23 例（63.89%）。≥2 cm 结石中 SRS 组 14 例（31.82%）为多发性结石，对照组为 2 例（14.29%）。

表 2　＜2 cm 结石和单发性≥2 cm 结石患者的手术时间比较 ($\bar{x}\pm s$)

组别	例数	结石直径＜2 cm			例数	单发性结石直径≥2 cm		
		结石直径（cm）	总手术时间（min）	结石清除时间（min）		结石直径（cm）	总手术时间（min）	结石清除时间（min）
SRS 组	30	1.39±0.31	46.81±15.00	8.83±10.58	30	3.21±1.02	54.07±19.57	21.93±16.72
对照组	36	0.98±0.40	62.51±25.43	28.95±27.49	12	2.46±0.45	79.85±24.63	43.28±24.18
t 值		4.562 6	2.513 9	3.719 7		0.486 5	3.531 2	3.251 9
P 值		＜0.001	＜0.02	＜0.001		＞0.05	＜0.01	＜0.01

2.3 ≥2 cm 结石组清除一枚结石所需手术时间

两组相比，清除一枚结石所需平均手术时间 SRS 组均少于对照组，差异有统计学意义（$P<0.001$）。

SRS 组<2 cm 结石患者的结石直径较大，其中 4 例直接用取石钳取出，其余 26 例碎石后取出。对照组<2 cm 结石中 4 例直接用 Ellick 冲吸器取出，15 例用电切襻取出，其余 16 例碎石后取出。≥2 cm 结石均需碎石后才能取出。

表 3 ≥2 cm 结石组清除一枚结石所需的手术时间　（$\bar{x}\pm s$）

项目	SRS 组	对照组	t 值	P 值
例数	44	14		
累计结石数（枚）	81	17		
平均结石数（个）	1.84±1.88	1.21±0.43	1.237 0	>0.05
结石直径（cm）	2.48±1.07	2.45±0.47	0.300 0	>0.05
手术时间（min）	12.84±14.04	33.23±25.26	4.650 6	<0.001

2.4 两组患者的并发症比较

对照组术中转开放手术 3 例（6.00％）。1 例直径 3.2 cm 结石，结构坚硬。结石无法用镜鞘固定，碎石时在膀胱腔内不断滑动，钬激光碎石效率无法发挥。改用输尿管镜直接碎石，由于不能持续冲洗手术视野模糊。手术进行 1 h 后发现膀胱黏膜损伤导致膀胱壁破裂；2 例由于碎石过多无法净。2 例 3 月后继发尿道狭窄。

SRS 组无特殊并发症发生，无中转开放手术。但是有 1 例 97 岁多发性结石，最大结石直径 5.8 cm，另一枚结石直径 2.2 cm，其余 15 枚结石<2 cm，为手术安全，碎石 102 min 后终止手术，2 周后再行碎石。另有 4 例患者伴有尿道狭窄或尿道内径过小，先行尿道扩张，改用 F24 电切镜行 TURP，然后碎石。此时，由于前列腺窝创面的渗血，手术视野较模糊。

3 讨论

现有腔内微创技术仅适用于直径<2 cm 的膀胱结石[12]，其主要原因是术中常遇到的 4 大难题：①膀胱空腔大，膀胱结石多而坚硬，碎石时容易在腔内滑动；②结石粉碎后形成大量碎石加之尿道弯曲，应用现有设备不易取出；③膀胱壁充盈后变薄，容易损伤穿孔；④无法继续冲洗，视野不清。

应用输尿管镜联合电切镜进行膀胱碎石是一种有效的方法[3]，但是镜鞘固定结石的稳定性远不如 SRS 系统的取石钳，结石过大时常无法固定结石。

碎石时结石经常在膀胱腔内不断滑动，钬激光碎石效率无法有效发挥。用输尿管镜直接碎石，由于输尿管镜进水流量小，又不能持续冲洗，手术视野常模糊不清，容易损伤膀胱黏膜。一旦黏膜损伤出血，视野将更加模糊。加之膀胱壁充盈后变薄，容易损伤穿孔。因此这种方法在处理较大结石时容易损伤膀胱黏膜导致膀胱壁破裂。术中细小结石可采用 Ellick 冲吸器冲吸，也可用电切襻在操作腔内或镜鞘外取出较大碎石。但是取石效率低，容易损坏电切襻。反复使用后容易损坏电切镜上用于锁定电切襻的固定器。本文 2 例由于碎石后产生过多碎石，无法彻底取净，最终改行开放手术。其次，经尿道反复插入电切镜取石会严重损伤尿道黏膜，可导致术后继发性尿道狭窄发生。因此这种方法更适用于直径<2 cm 的结石。

SRS 系统是一种金属硬性内镜。取石钳位于物镜的前端，由上向下张合，钳床闭合时纵观呈圆形，其中央部依为圆形腔道。取石钳夹片为框架状，在碎石时易于抓取、固定结石。钳夹的顶端边缘设有阻挡襻后可在镜鞘内进行拖网式取石，一次可取出多枚结石。金属钳夹可有力地控制 6.4 cm 以下的结石进行碎石操作。镜鞘也可与冲吸器相连冲洗结石。应用流体力学回旋流原理，带有出水孔的镜鞘使 SRS 系统具有自动收集结石的功能。碎石通道位于物镜和光源的下缘，便于在直视下抓取结石进行碎石操作。

术中 SRS 系统可在直视下入镜，结石固定后再进行碎石操作，此时结石无法再在膀胱腔内滑动，用钬激光或气压弹道碎石时碎石效率大幅提高，结石容易粉碎。其次，SRS 系统具有连续冲洗功能，进、出水流量大。因此术中可保持清晰视野，便于操作，不易损伤膀胱黏膜。结石粉碎后用 SRS 系统的取石钳在镜鞘内拖网式取石，一次可取出多枚碎石。有较多细小碎石时也可采用冲吸器冲吸取石。同时 SRS 系统的镜鞘内径远大于 F26 连续冲洗型 Storze 电切镜的操作内径，可取出更大碎石。这样可明显提高取石效率，缩短手术时间。不同于电切镜的电切襻取石方法，SRS 系统的取石钳取石操作一般都是在镜鞘内进行，这样可有效减少镜鞘反复插入尿道导致的尿道黏膜损伤。

为避免意外损伤，SRS 系统镜鞘置入膀胱后应直视下插入取石钳。较大结石可以在镜鞘外直接取出，但这样的操作对尿道黏膜损伤大，不宜反复使用。术中保持低压持续冲洗可保持视野清晰、避免膀胱黏膜损伤。我们推荐碎石后再行 TURP，这样更易操作。对于高龄、高危、结石体积过大和数目过多的患者，可采用分期碎石治疗。

95

440   J Mod Urol, Vol. 18 No. 5 Sep. 2013

总之,SRS 系统是一种集固定结石、提供碎石通道、自动收集碎石、摄取碎石、冲吸碎石和连续冲洗等功能为一体的多功能内镜。尤其是术中可固定结石、自动收集碎石、一次可摄取多枚碎石。这样可缩短手术时间,提高碎石效率,拓展内镜治疗膀胱结石的手术适应范围。其联合 TURP 用于治疗膀胱结石伴 BPH 是一种安全、有效的治疗方法,但临床病例有待进一步积累。

参考文献:

[1] WONG M. Bladder calculi, an evidence-based review[M]. In: Stone disease. The 2nd International Consultation on Stone Disease. Paris: Editions 21, 2008, 295-303.

[2] DHABALIA JV, JAIN N, KUMAR V, et al. Modified technique of percutaneous cystolithotripsy using a new instrument-combined single-step trocar-dilator with self-retaining adjustable access sheath[J]. Urology, 2011, 77(6): 1304-1307.

[3] TUGCU V, POLAT H, OZBAY B, et al. Percutaneous versus transurethral cystolithotripsy[J]. J Endourol, 2009, 23(2): 237-241.

[4] ELCIOGLU O, OZDEN H, GUVEN G, et al. Urinary bladder stone extraction and instruments compared in textbooks of Abul-Qasim Khalaf Ibn Abbas Alzahrawi (Albucasis) (930-1013) and Serefeddin Sabuncuoglu (1385-1470)[J]. J Endourol, 2010, 24 (9): 1463-1468.

[5] SINGH KJ, KAURL J. Comparison of three different endoscopic techniques in management of bladder calculi[J]. Indian J Urol, 2011, 27(1): 10-13.

[6] ENER K, AGRAS K, ALDEMIR M, et al. The randomized comparison of two different endoscopic techniques in the management of large bladder stones: transurethral use of nephroscope or cystoscope?[J]. J Endourol, 2009, 23(7): 1151-1155.

[7] KARA C, RESORLU B, CICEKBILEK I, et al. Transurethral cystolithotripsy with holmium laser under local anesthesia in selected patients[J]. Urology, 2009, 74(5): 1000-1003.

[8] PHILIPPOU P, VOLANIS D, KARIOTIS I, et al. Prospective comparative study of endoscopic management of bladder lithiasis: is prostate surgery a necessary adjunct?[J]. Urology, 2011, 78(1): 43-47.

[9] SHAH HN, HEGDE SS, SHAH JN, et al. Simultaneous transurethral cystolithotripsy with holmium laser enucleation of the prostate: a prospective feasibility study and review of literature [J]. BJU Int, 2007, 99(3): 595-600.

[10] LI A, LU H, LIU S, et al. A Novel Endoscope to Treat Bladder stone[J]. J Endourol Part B (Videourology), 2011, 25: doi: 10. 1089.

[11] LI A, JI C, LU H, et al. Transurethral cystolithotripsy with a novel special endoscope[J]. Urol Res, 2012, 40(6): 769-773.

[12] 夏术阶. 膀胱结石碎石术[M]//夏术阶. 微创泌尿外科学. 济南: 山东科学技术出版社, 2007: 143-144.

(编辑　何宏灵)

(上接第 430 页)

本研究发现 miR-154 对于细胞周期的影响非常明显,我们下一步针对 miR-154 可能调节的细胞周期蛋白进行研究,分析其抑制前列腺癌细胞增殖的具体作用机制,并结合临床资料如 PSA、fPSA、Gleason 评分及随访资料,以期找到 miR-154 调控的具体机制或相关通路,发现前列腺癌可能的分子诊断标志和干预靶点。

综上所述,本研究结果提示,在前列腺癌中 miR-154 的表达下降,而上调 miR-154 可以使前列腺癌细胞阻滞在 G_1 期,而抑制细胞的增殖,因此 miR-154 可以影响前列腺癌细胞的增殖能力,有望成为前列腺癌治疗的新靶点。

参考文献:

[1] LAI EC. Micro RNAs are complementary to 3'UTR sequence motifs that mediate negative post-transcriptional regulation[J]. Nat Genet 2002, 30: 363-364.

[2] BARTEL DP. MicroRNAs: Genomics, biogenesis, mechanism, and function[J]. Cell, 2004, 116, 281-297.

[3] SZCZYRBA J, LÖPRICH E, WACH S, et al. The micro RNA profile of prostate carcinoma obtained by deep sequencing[J]. Mol Cancer Res, 2010, 8: 529-538.

[4] FILIPOWICZ W, GROSSHANS H. The liver-specific microRNA miR-122: biology and therapeutic potential[J]. Prog Drug Res, 2011, 67: 221-238.

[5] ABRAHAM D, JACKSON N, GUNDARA JS, et al. MicroRNA profiling of sporadic and hereditary medullary thyroid cancer identifies predictors of nodal metastasis, prognosis, and potential therapeutic targets[J]. Clin Cancer Res, 2011, 17: 4772-4781.

[6] WANG W, PENG B, WANG D, et al. Human tumor microRNA signatures derived from large-scale oligonucleotide microarray datasets[J]. Int J Cancer, 2011, 129, 1624-1634.

[7] JEMAL A, SIEGEL R, WARD E, et al. Cancer statis-tics, 2009 [J]. CA Cancer J Clin, 2009, 59: 225-249.

[8] YANG L, PARKIN DM, FERLAY J, et al. Estimates of cancer incidence in China for 2000 and projections for 2005[J]. Cancer Epidemiol Biomarkers Prev, 2005, 14(1): 243-250.

(编辑　何宏灵)

附录 3
国际会议发言交流证书

1. 国际泌尿外科学会第 31 届大会视频发言交流证书

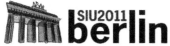

Aihua Li

31st CONGRESS of the SOCIÉTÉ INTERNATIONALE D'UROLOGIE
ICC BERLIN ▶ October 16-20 ▶ 2011

CERTIFICATE OF PRESENTATION

This document certifies that

Aihua Li
Binghui Zhang
Honghai Lu
Sikuan Liu
Feng Zhang
Xiaoqiang Qian
Hui Wang
Wei Fang

presented

AH-1 Stone Removal System to Treat Bladder Stones

as a

Video Presentation

at the 31st Congress of the SIU in Berlin, Germany
held October 16-20, 2011.

We would like to thank all of our presenters for contributing to
the success of this year's scientific programme.

Gerald H. Jordan, MD
Chair, Scientific Programme Committee
31st SIU Congress

Michael Marberger, MD
Co-Chair, Scientific Programme Committee
31st SIU Congress

2. 国际泌尿外科学会第 35 届大会第 4 届泌尿外科先进适宜新技术论坛发言推广交流证书

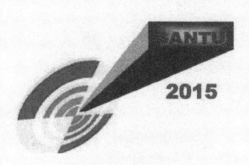

The 4th Symposium on Affordable New Technologies in Urology

Organized during the

35th Congress of the Societé Internationale d'Urologie

October 15th, 2015 at the Melbourne Congress & Exhibition Centre, Melbourne - Australia

POSTER PRESENTER CERTIFICATE

This is to Confirm That

Aihua Li from **China** presented a Poster on

Transurethral Cystolitholapaxy with the AH-1 Stone Removal System to Treat Large Volume Bladder Stones

Prof. Daniel Yachia

Honorary Chairman

Dr. Lukman Hakim

Chairman

3. 第 34 届世界腔道泌尿外科大会发言交流邀请函

Notice of Paper Abstract Acceptance, WCE 2016: Congratulations!

发件人：　**smevorach** <smevorach@urologymanagement.org>

收件人：　li121288@aliyun.com <li121288@aliyun.com>

抄　送：　maillog <maillog@ConferenceHarvester.com>

时　间：　2016年8月12日(星期五) 07:43

11 August 2016

Dear Aihua Li,

We are pleased to inform you that your paper abstract(s):

199222 : Efficiency of Transurethral Cystolitholapaxy with AH -1 Stone Removal System to Large Volume Bladder Stones

199813 : The Efficiency of Transurethral Resection and Degeneration of Bladder Tumor to Treat Bladder Cancer　A 10 Year Review

has been accepted for presentation in a "Moderated Poster Session" at the 2016 World Congress of Endourology, taking place 8 - 12 November 2016 in Cape Town, South Africa.

To access the online portal and accept or decline this invitation, register for the meeting, complete all necessary tasks as well as access information about printing your poster and presenting at the Congress, please log in to your portal below:

WORLD CONGRESS OF ENDOUROLOGY - PAPER & VIDEO ABSTRACTS SITE

URL: https://www.ConferenceHarvester.com/harvester2/login.asp?EventKey=HISJNODX

Username: li121288@aliyun.com

Password (Access Key): K Z J V A A U G

You must accept or decline this invitation no later than **August 29**. If we do not receive a response on or before this date, we will assume that you will present this abstract at the World Congress of Endourology in Cape Town, South Africa. All tasks in the portal must be completed before the deadlines.

SESSION INFORMATION: All moderated poster session dates and times will be announced in a follow-up email in the coming week.

As a presenting author, it is your responsibility to notify other authors/colleagues that this abstract has been accepted.

Reminder: All authors making presentations are required to disclose any financial support from, or business affiliation with, industry in connection with any product or technique reported in their presentations. This disclosure is to be clearly and prominently displayed on your poster.

If you have been accepted for more than one presentation format, you will receive a separate email. If you have any questions, please contact Saroyah Mevorach, smevorach@urologymanagement.org for assistance.

Thank you for your participation and congratulations! We look forward to seeing you in Cape Town.

Sincerely yours,

Margaret S. Pearle, MD, PhD.

Secretary General

Endourological Society

Marius Conradie

President

2016 World Congress of Endourology

Andre van der Merwe

Secretary

2016 World Congress of Endourology

附录 4

授权专利证书

1. 膀胱肾盂取石镜

国际发明专利(PCT)WO2009／092182282

102

2. 膀胱肾盂取石镜
发明专利 ZL2008132850.4

证书号 第698971号

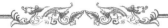

发明专利证书

发 明 名 称：膀胱肾盂取石镜

发　明　人：李爱华

专　利　号：ZL 2008 1 0032850.4

专利申请日：2008 年 01 月 21 日

专利权人：上海市杨浦区中心医院

授权公告日：2010 年 11 月 10 日

　　本发明经过本局依照中华人民共和国专利法进行审查，决定授予专利权，颁发本证书并在专利登记簿上予以登记。专利权自授权公告之日起生效。

　　本专利的专利权期限为二十年，自申请日起算。专利权人应当依照专利法及其实施细则规定缴纳年费。本专利的年费应在每年01月21日前缴纳。未按照规定缴纳年费的，专利权自应当缴纳年费期满之日起终止。

　　专利证书记载专利权登记时的法律状况。专利权的转移、质押、无效、终止、恢复和专利权人的姓名或名称、国籍、地址变更等事项记载在专利登记簿上。

局长 田力普

2010 年 11 月 10 日

第 1 页（共 1 页）

3. 用于膀胱肾盂取石镜的钳夹
实用新型专利 ZL200820054918.4

证 书 号 第1165889号

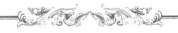

实用新型专利证书

实用新型名称：用于膀胱肾盂取石镜的钳夹

发　明　人：李爱华

专　利　号：ZL 2008 2 0054918.4

专利申请日：2008年1月21日

专 利 权 人：上海市杨浦区中心医院

授权公告日：2009年1月21日

　　本实用新型经过本局依照中华人民共和国专利法进行初步审查，决定授予专利权，颁发本证书并在专利登记簿上予以登记。专利权自授权公告之日起生效。

　　本专利的专利权期限为十年，自申请日起算。专利权人应当依照专利法及其实施细则规定缴纳年费。缴纳本专利年费的期限是每年1月21日前一个月内。未按照规定缴纳年费的，专利权自应当缴纳年费期满之日起终止。

　　专利证书记载专利权登记时的法律状况。专利权的转移、质押、无效、终止、恢复和专利权人的姓名或名称、国籍、地址变更等事项记载在专利登记簿上。

局长 田力普

2009年1月21日

第 1 页（共 1 页）

4. 冲洗结构改良型膀胱肾盂取石镜
实用新型专利 ZL200820155132.1

证 书 号第1268622号

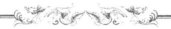

实用新型专利证书

实用新型名称: 冲洗结构改良型膀胱肾盂取石镜

发　明　人: 李爱华

专　利　号: ZL 2008 2 0155132.1

专利申请日: 2008年11月10日

专利权人: 上海市杨浦区中心医院

授权公告日: 2009年8月12日

　　本实用新型经过本局依照中华人民共和国专利法进行初步审查，决定授予专利权，颁发本证书并在专利登记簿上予以登记，专利权自授权公告之日起生效。

　　本专利的专利权期限为十年，自申请日起算。专利权人应当依照专利法及其实施细则规定缴纳年费。缴纳本专利年费的期限是每年11月10日前一个月内。未按照规定缴纳年费的，专利权自应当缴纳年费期满之日起终止。

　　专利证书记载专利权登记时的法律状况。专利权的转移、质押、无效、终止、恢复和专利权人的姓名或名称、国籍、地址变更等事项记载在专利登记簿上。

局长　田力普

2009年8月12日

第 1 页 (共 1 页)

5. 镜鞘壁上设有出水孔的膀胱肾盂取石镜
实用新型专利 ZL200920072709.7

证书号第1465446号

实用新型专利证书

实用新型名称：镜鞘鞘壁上设有出水孔的膀胱肾盂取石镜

发　明　人：李爱华

专　利　号：ZL 2009 2 0072709.7

专利申请日：2009 年 05 月 21 日

专 利 权 人：上海市杨浦区中心医院

授权公告日：2010 年 06 月 23 日

　　本实用新型经过本局依照中华人民共和国专利法进行初步审查，决定授予专利权，颁发本证书并在专利登记簿上予以登记。专利权自授权公告之日起生效。

　　本专利的专利权期限为十年，自申请日起算。专利权人应当依照专利法及其实施细则规定缴纳年费。本专利的年费应当在每年 05 月 21 日前缴纳。未按照规定缴纳年费的，专利权自应当缴纳年费期满之日起终止。

　　专利证书记载专利权登记时的法律状况。专利权的转移、质押、无效、终止、恢复和专利权人的姓名或名称、国籍、地址变更等事项记载在专利登记簿上。

局长 田力普

2010 年 06 月 23 日

第 1 页 （共 1 页）

6. 用于膀胱肾盂取石镜的镜桥
实用新型专利 ZL201220007532.4

证书号 第2392323号

实用新型专利证书

实用新型名称：用于膀胱肾盂取石镜的镜桥

发　明　人：李爱华

专　利　号：ZL. 2012 2 0007532.4

专利申请日：2012 年 01 月 10 日

专利权人：上海市杨浦区中心医院

授权公告日：2012 年 09 月 05 日

　　本实用新型经过本局依照中华人民共和国专利法进行初步审查，决定授予专利权，颁发本证书并在专利登记簿上予以登记。专利权自授权公告之日起生效。

　　本专利的专利权期限为十年，自申请日起算。专利权人应当依照专利法及其实施细则规定缴纳年费。本专利的年费应当在每年 01 月 10 日前缴纳。未按照规定缴纳年费的，专利权自应当缴纳年费期满之日起终止。

　　专利证书记载专利权登记时的法律状况。专利权的转移、质押、无效、终止、恢复和专利权人的姓名或名称、国籍、地址变更等事项记载在专利登记簿上。

局长　田力普

2012 年 09 月 05 日

第 1 页（共 1 页）

7. 用于膀胱肾盂取石镜的多用途镜鞘转换器
实用新型专利 ZL201520141769.5

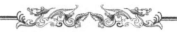

证 书 号 第 4474069 号

实用新型专利证书

实用新型名称：用于膀胱肾盂取石镜的镜鞘转换器

发 明 人：李爱华

专 利 号：ZL 2015 2 0141769.5

专利申请日：2015 年 03 月 12 日

专 利 权 人：上海市杨浦区中心医院

授权公告日：2015 年 07 月 29 日

　　本实用新型经过本局依照中华人民共和国专利法进行初步审查，决定授予专利权，颁发本证书并在专利登记簿上予以登记，专利权自授权公告之日起生效。

　　本专利的专利权期限为十年，自申请日起算。专利权人应当依照专利法及其实施细则规定缴纳年费。本专利的年费应当在每年 03 月 12 日前缴纳。未按照规定缴纳年费的，专利权自应当缴纳年费期满之日起终止。

　　专利证书记载专利权登记时的法律状况。专利权的转移、质押、无效、终止、恢复和专利权人的姓名或名称、国籍、地址变更等事项记载在专利登记簿上。

局长
申长雨

2015 年 07 月 29 日

第 1 页 (共 1 页)

附录 5
学术奖励证书

1. 2010 年获上海医学科技三等奖证书

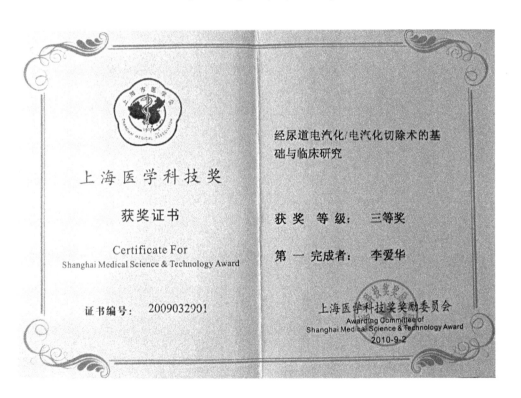

上海市医学协会

上海医学科技奖

获奖证书

Certificate For
Shanghai Medical Science & Technology Award

证书编号： 2009032901

经尿道电汽化/电汽化切除术的基础与临床研究

获 奖 等 级： 三等奖

第 一 完成者： 李爱华

上海医学科技奖奖励委员会
Awarding Committee of
Shanghai Medical Science & Technology Award
2010-9-2

2. 2012 年获第二十四届上海市优秀发明选拔赛
职工技术创新成果铜奖证书

3. 2013 年入围吴阶平泌尿外科医学奖网页

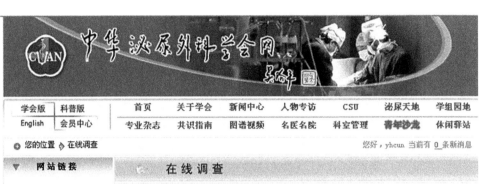

中华泌尿外科学会网

| 学会版 | 科普版 | 首页 | 关于学会 | 新闻中心 | 人物专访 | CSU | 泌尿天地 | 学组园地 |
| English | 会员中心 | 专业杂志 | 共识指南 | 图谱视频 | 名医名院 | 科室管理 | 青年沙龙 | 休闲驿站 |

◉ 您的位置 ◈ 在线调查　　　　　　　　　　　您好，yhcun 当前有 0 条新消息

▼　**网站链接**

在线调查

Google Translate
Select Language ▾
✚ Google　Gadgets powered by Google

2013年吴阶平泌尿外科医学奖评选

候选人列表（左键点击投票框，最多选择5人）

☐ 李虹　四川大学华西医院

☐ 沈周俊　上海交通大学医学院附属瑞金医院

☐ 程跃　宁波市第一医院

☐ 谢立平　浙江大学医学院附属第一医院

☐ 梁朝朝　安徽医科大学第一附属医院

☐ 文建国　郑州大学第一附属医院

☐ 马潞林　北京大学第三医院

☐ 李开弟　内蒙鄂尔多斯市卫校附属医院

☐ 王东文　山西医科大学第一医院

☐ 潘铁军　广州军区武汉总医院

候选项目列表（左键点击投票框，最多选择2项）

☐ CTA引导下肾段动脉精确阻断腹腔镜肾部分切除术的应用　南京医科大学第一附属医院泌尿外科

☐ 计算机模拟训练在泌尿外科内镜培训中的应用研究　中国泌尿外科学院、北京大学吴阶平泌尿外科医学中心、北京大学首钢医院

☑ AH-1型取石系统的研制和临床应用　同济大学附属杨浦医院（上海市杨浦区中心医院）

☐ 中国商环包皮环切术在农村的推广价值　宁波大学附属宁波市第一医院

☐ 基于CT胶片的腹膜后腔个体化三维模型及手术导引系统的构建与应用　山西医科大学第一医院泌尿外科

提交

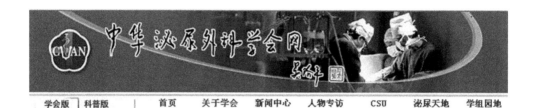

| 学会版 | 科普版 | 首页 | 关于学会 | 新闻中心 | 人物专访 | CSU | 泌尿天地 | 学组园地 |
| English | 会员中心 | 专业杂志 | 共识指南 | 图谱视频 | 名医名院 | 科室管理 | 青年沙龙 | 休闲驿站 |

◈ 您的位置：专业版首页 ◈ 新闻中心

▼ RSS 频道

XML RSS 2.0

RSS频道订阅帮助

▼ 网站链接

Google Translate
Select Language ▼
Google Gadgets powered by Google

🐾 新闻中心

关于CUA委员投票推选2013年吴阶平泌尿外科医学奖的通告

2013年吴阶平泌尿外科医学奖初评工作于2013年7月8日起在CUA网站开始进行，截止7月31日，获得个人前五名的是（按姓氏笔画排序）北京大学第三医院马潞林、山西医科大学第一医院王东文、四川大学华西医院李虹、浙江大学医学院附属第一医院谢立平、广州军区武汉总医院潘铁军，获得项目前五名的是计算机模拟训练在泌尿外科内镜培训中的应用研究、中国商环包皮环切术在农村的推广价值、基于CT胶片的腹膜后腔个体化三维模型及手术导引系统的构建与应用、CTA引导下肾段动脉精确阻断腹腔镜肾部分切除术的应用、AH-1型取石系统的研制和临床应用。

现向第九届CUA全国委员征求选票。

规则：1）每张选票只能选择3名个人和3个项目；

2）请于2013年11月15日17:00前将选票发往CUA网站编辑部 editor@cuan.cn ，逾期失效。

3）个人资料和项目介绍请参阅《2013年吴阶平泌尿外科医学奖候选人及项目介绍》

CUA 网站
2013年10月30日

点击此处下载选票

4. 2014 年度上海市技术发明三等奖证书

上海市科学技术奖

证 书

为表彰上海市技术发明奖获得者，特颁发此证书。

项目名称：AH-1型取石系统的研制和临床转化

获 奖 者：李爱华

奖励等级：三等奖

上海市人民政府
2014年11月26日

证书号：20143020-3-R01

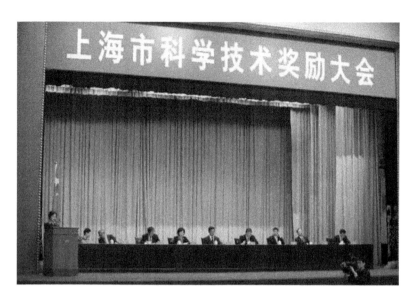

2014 年度上海市科学技术奖励大会

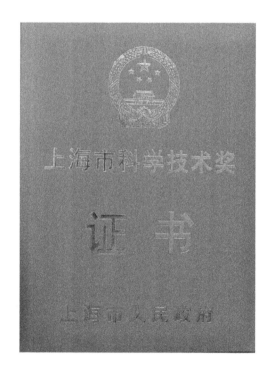

5. 2015 年度华夏医学科技奖三等奖

华夏医学科技奖
证　书

为表彰华夏医学科技奖获得者，特颁发此证书。

项目名称：AH-1型多功能取石系统的研制和在经尿道膀胱碎石术中的应用

获奖等级：三等奖

获 奖 者：李爱华

2015年11月29日

证书号：201503092P0801

附录 6
国际诊疗指南书籍 *Stone Disease* 引用推荐页面

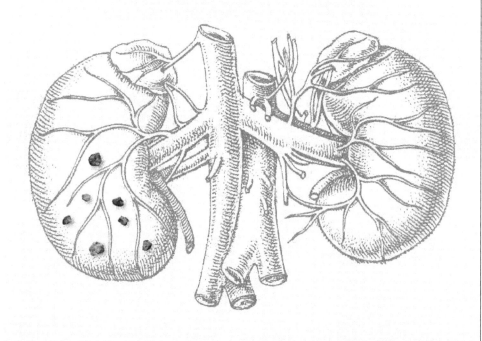

STONE DISEASE

EDITORS: John Denstedt, MD and Jean de la Rosette, MD

A Joint SIU-ICUD International Consultation

Glasgow, Scotland, October 12–15, 2014

Co-sponsored by
SIU (Société Internationale d'Urologie)
ICUD (International Consultation on Urological Diseases)

A number of lithotripters have been employed for stone fragmentation, including mechanical, electrohydraulic, pneumatic, ultrasonic, and Holmium laser.[27-36] Razvi *et al.*[28] compared the safety and efficacy of mechanical, ultrasonic, electrohydraulic, and Lithoclast lithotripters. They reported that devices such as ultrasound (U/S) or pneumatic lithotripters may utilize larger, rigid probes, and may be more efficient for patients with large or hard stones. Un-no *et al.*[29] compared Holmium:yttrium aluminum garnet (YAG) laser to Swiss Lithoclast. They concluded that both lithotripters are safe and effective to fragment stones at one session. However, Holmium:YAG laser is preferable for the fragmentation and removal of the fragment in large bladder stones. In general, Holmium:YAG laser has been employed with success for large bladder calculi (>5 cm) with minimal morbidity.[30,31] Its efficacy and safety was proved for the management of bladder lithiasis secondary to renal transplantation, as well.[36] Recently, a novel stone removal system was introduced for the fragmentation of bladder stones. This system is comprised of a jaw, utilized for stone fixation and for fragments removal, and a tube through which the laser fiber or pneumatic lithotripter probe can be inserted. First results in 35 patients showed that this system can decrease significantly the operation time compared to Holmium laser.[37]

TABLE 8-2 Studies Evaluating Transurethral Cystolithotripsy

	Patients, n	Lithotripter type	SFR, %	LOE	GOR
Razvi *et al.*[28]	106	Mech vs. EHL vs. U/S vs. Lithoclast	90 vs. 63 vs. 88 vs. 85	3	C
Teichman *et al.*[30]	14	Holmium	100	3	C
Grasso[31]	63	Holmium	97	3	C
Asci *et al.*[32]	93	Mech vs. Mech+TURP	94 vs. 93	3	C
Shah *et al.*[33]	32	Holmium	100	3	C
Chtourou *et al.*[34]	120	Ballistic	97.5	3	C
Sinik *et al.*[35]	52	Pneumatic	100	3	C
Li *et al.*[37]	35	AH-1 vs. Holmium	97.1 vs. 78.6	3	C

AH-1, Aihua-1 stone removal system; EHL, electrohydraulic lithotripter; mech, mechanical lithotripter; TURP, transurethral resection of the prostate; U/S, ultrasonic lithotripter.

8.1.4.3　Percutaneous cystolithotripsy

Spare the implication of urethra and bladder neck while retrieving with bladder stones is appealing. In general, stones >4 cm are considered unsuitable for transurethral cystolithotripsy, with the exception of Holmium laser modality.[30,31] Percutaneous techniques have implemented lately for the management of large calculi mainly as an alternative to open techniques. Stone-free rates are excellent, reported to be between 89% and 100%.[38-40] Ultrasonic, mechanic, or pneumatic lithotripter may be used for stone fragmentation (**Table 8-3**). History of bladder cancer, previous abdominal surgery, and radiation to the pelvis may represent a contraindication.

There are only two studies to directly compare percutaneous technique with transurethral cystolithotripsy in patients who undergo a simultaneous prostate removal. Aron *et al.*[41] reported that percutaneous technique is safe, more effective, and a much faster alternative to a transurethral one,